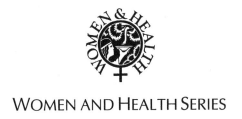

# WOMEN AND HEALTH SERIES

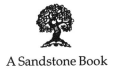

A Sandstone Book

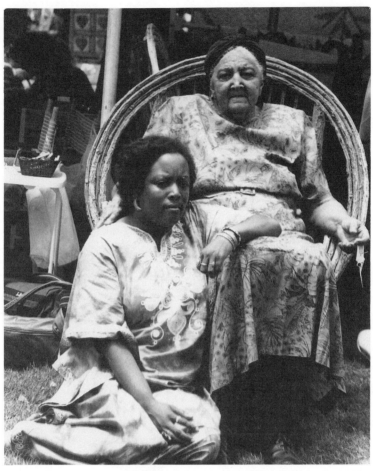

Linda Janet Holmes and Margaret Charles Smith after Talking Tent, Birmingham, 1993. Photo by William Dickey.

# LISTEN TO ME GOOD
## The Life Story of
## an Alabama Midwife

Margaret Charles Smith
*and* Linda Janet Holmes

*A Helen Hooven Santmyer Prize Winner*

OHIO STATE UNIVERSITY PRESS
COLUMBUS

**Library of Congress Cataloging-in-Publication Data**

Smith, Margaret Charles, 1906–
    Listen to me good : the life story of an Alabama midwife /
Margaret Charles Smith and Linda Janet Holmes.
        p.   cm.   — (Women and health series)
    "A  Helen Hooven Santmyer Prize winner"
    Includes bibliographical references and index.
        ISBN 0-8142-0700-6 (cloth : alk. paper).   — ISBN 0-8142-0701-4
(paper : alk. paper)
        1. Smith, Margaret Charles, 1906–   .  2. Afro-American midwives—
Alabama—Eutaw—Biography.  3. Midwifery—Alabama—Eutaw—
History. I. Holmes, Linda Janet, 1949–  . II. Title.  III. Series: Women &
health (Columbus, Ohio)
    RG962.E98S65   1996
    618.2'0233—dc20
    [b]                                                                                               96-15037
                                                                                                           CIP

Text, jacket, and cover design by Donna Hartwick.
Jacket and cover photo by William Dickey.
Type set in Palatino and Optima.
Printed by Braun-Brumfield, Inc., Ann Arbor, Michigan.

The paper in this publication meets the minimum requirements of American
National Standard for Information Sciences—Permanence of Paper for Printed
Library Materials. ANSI 239.48-1992.

9   8   7   6   5   4   3   2

*To Alabama midwives—with respect*

—M. C. S.

*For Toni Cade Bambara, 1939–1995*

—L. J. H.

Three dollars cash
For a pair of catalog shoes
Was what the midwife charged
My Mama
For bringing me

———————

—ALICE WALKER, *"Three Dollars Cash"*

# CONTENTS

# SERIES EDITORS' PREFACE

*Together Margaret Charles Smith* and Linda Janet Holmes have brought us the gifts of plain and honest talk and of thoughtful and powerful history. Mrs. Smith describes with grace and power her life and work as a midwife in Alabama's Greene County. In her autobiography, she remembers births like the one that took place in a house with a pig in one corner and a goat in another. She tells of birthing customs that will soon be forgotten, like using mayapple-root tea to stop premature labor. And she recalls the rural poverty and racial segregation when black people toiled for a dollar a day and sat at the back of the bus. But Mrs. Smith does not dwell in the past; she focuses on the contemporary political situation and voices fears about AIDS. As we read, we find her voice becoming a friend's—the voice of someone we trust to tell us the truth.

Linda Janet Holmes not only listened to Mrs. Smith's story; she has recorded and presented it with great knowledge and sensitivity. She is our guide, mapping Mrs. Smith's community for us, walking us through the streets of Eutaw. She points to the places where civil rights demonstrators gathered, and she journeys with us to Tuskegee to show us where Mrs. Smith underwent some of her training. Together with Mrs. Smith, Linda Janet Holmes welcomes us to Eutaw and lets us understand the many lessons to be learned there.

We are proud to have *Listen to Me Good* in the Women and Health Series of the Ohio State University Press, and we are pleased to introduce this autobiography to our readers.

# ACKNOWLEDGMENTS

*In 1981 an independent fellowship* from the National Endowment for the Humanities supported me during a year's research on southern black midwifery. The University of Medicine and Dentistry of New Jersey's Nurse-Midwife Educational Program, along with an anonymous New England donor, assisted in the initial transcription of the interviews of midwives I collected. West Alabama Health Services in Eutaw, Greene County, contributed timely financial support along with advice and encouragement. James Coleman, the executive director, Sandral Hullett, the medical director, and Para Davis, a special assistant at West Alabama, showed an unwavering commitment to this book. The photographers Sharon Blackmon, William Dickey, and Charles Robertson donated several illustrations.

Many people read early drafts or excerpts of this work and provided valuable feedback. I thank Joan Burstyn, Libby Cousins, Mindy Fullilove, David Koester, Sandral Hullett, Jane Pincus, Alonzo Speight, and Charles Robertson. I am very grateful to Carol Vance of Columbia University Graduate School of Public Health for her probing criticisms. Many of my classmates at Columbia encouraged this work, but Pamela Peterside-Browne stands out for her support when it seemed doubtful that the book would ever see the light of day. Both Charlotte Dihoff and Janet Golden knew what to say and do to keep this book moving toward publication.

I am also thankful for friends whose influences simply floated through me into the work. Several people exercised their personal magic. Toni Cade Bambara, my mentor when I was an undergraduate at Rutgers University and lifelong friend, hears my calls whenever I take walks in the woods or pick up shells on the beach. Other positive influences either dropped their inspiration gently like morning dew or struck like lightning. Thanks to Byllye Avery, Marie Browne, Pepsi Charles, Robin Foster Drain, Tom Feelings, Judy Funches, Obery Hendricks, Peggy Horan, Deborah Horsley, Jane Kerina, Ken O'Dowd, Indu Krishnan, Judy Litoff, Louie Massiah, Sheryl Ruzek, Beverly Guy-Sheftal, Welton Smith, Joan Whitlow, and the late Gerri Wilson.

In the final stage of my research, my Alabama safety net was key. Some of the people who opened doors, welcomed me to eat, and provided a place to sleep are Charlotte Borst, Sharon Blackmon, Charles Mauldin, Gwen Patton, Charles Robertson, and Sandral Hullett. My special love goes to Mrs. Leola Robertson, my Alabama mother, and her daughter, Khadijah (Sylvia Robertson), who first invited me to Selma in the summer of 1971.

In New Jersey, my New Hope Baptist Church family grounded me in prayer. At New Hope, the Rev. Charles E. Thomas, an Alabama native, continues to inspire with the stories of growing up in Montgomery that he tells in his sermons. On the very day after I was baptized at New Hope, I received the fellowship that allowed me to begin my work in Alabama. Now, during Communion at New Hope, I stare at the cross in the church window and see a midwife, Rosie Aaron Smith, who died in 1994 in Lowndesboro, Alabama. She taught me how to see spirits rising up in storms and moved me to get down on my knees and pray by the side of a Lowndes County road in broad daylight after I interviewed her.

My parents, Robert and Ann Holmes, and my sister,

Mary Ann, and her family, the Cools—Billy, Tumba, Malakhi, and Zetta—always kept a lookout for me. Occasionally they insisted that I come out of the world of Alabama midwives into the world of their ever-present love. Aunts, uncles, and cousins in New Jersey, Kentucky, and elsewhere strengthen me in my calling every time they tell me to keep writing.

Most important, I am grateful for my daughter, Ghana Smith. Only she knows how many New Year's resolutions, how much family time, and how much deep moaning I have put into trying to finish the book. When I fall into despair, she always assures me that all is well and helps me find the peace of mind to continue. Ghana deserves all the appreciation I can muster.

*Linda Janet Holmes*

*I want to thank* Laura Kate Smith. There's nobody on that hill now but her. She will carry me if I have to go to the doctor. If I want to get anywhere, she will carry me.

I want to thank Charles Robertson. He's such a sweet person. I love him to death. He enlightens you so much in his talking. Charles talks so much. Tells you things to do. He makes you feel like you are going to be happy. I gave up on this book a few times. Sometimes I got to the place where I felt the book just wasn't going to do no good nohow. But it wouldn't last long. See, Charles always said something good to help you make it.

Dr. Hullett, you know she went out of the way to help us. She sent Para Davis on her work time. We be gone half the day at a time, going round to different people getting information for the book. Para carried me a lot of places. We have to give Dr. Hullett and Para Davis praise for helping. For God's sake, we can't forget them.

## Acknowledgments

A whole lot of folks, some of them have passed, took a lot of time with me working at the clinic. But only one person went out with me on a birth. That was one time, and it was Alice Foreman. She was the nurse-midwife. One of the doctors I worked with a long time was Dr. Joe P. Smith. He is no longer living. They say he lost his mind before he died, but Dr. Smith, he was just plain-speaking. Whatever he tells you, it would come to pass. And in later years, it was Dr. Staggers who stood behind me until the end. Some of the other people I can think to thank are Christine Bell, Ernestelle Durrett, and Miss Hattie Atkins. Miss Hattie is no longer living. And I need to thank Barbara Tuck who worked at the clinic. Now she runs the secondhand store. She always was nice to me. Now Olla Mae Nixon, we were close friends. And Anita Davis with the WIC has always been nice to me. And Miss Margaret Cross the secretary, she took a lot of time with me. They were all nice people. I sure do want to thank them. But time come to be a midwife, I did that by myself.

*Margaret Charles Smith*

# CHRONOLOGY

## Life of Margaret Charles Smith

| | |
|---|---|
| 1906 (Sept. 12) | *Margaret Charles born in Eutaw.* |
| 1922 | *Son Houston born.* |
| 1926 | *Son Spencer born.* |
| c. 1939 | *Grandmother, born c. 1838, dies.* |
| 1942 | *Margaret Charles marries Randolph Smith.* |
| 1943 | *Son Herman born.* |
| 1949 | *Mrs. Smith obtains midwife permit, begins work at clinic.* |
| 1955 (Dec. 1) | *Rosa Parks arrested for refusing to give her seat to a white man. Montgomery bus boycott begins.* |
| 1963 (June 11) | *Gov. Wallace stands in doorway to block integration at the University of Alabama.* |
| 1965 (March 7) | *Bloody Sunday in Selma.* |
| 1965 (June) | *Protests shut down Tishibe clinic.* |
| 1966 | *Greene County Hospital opens.* |
| c. 1967 | *Randolph Smith, Mrs. Smith's husband, dies.* |
| 1969 | *Greene County elects first black slate; massive celebration at the courthouse. (Original courthouse was burned down by white vigilantes in 1867.)* |
| 1974 | *West Alabama Health Services opens.* |
| 1976 | *Nurse-midwife law outlaws lay midwives.* |
| 1981 | *Mrs. Smith attends last birth.* |

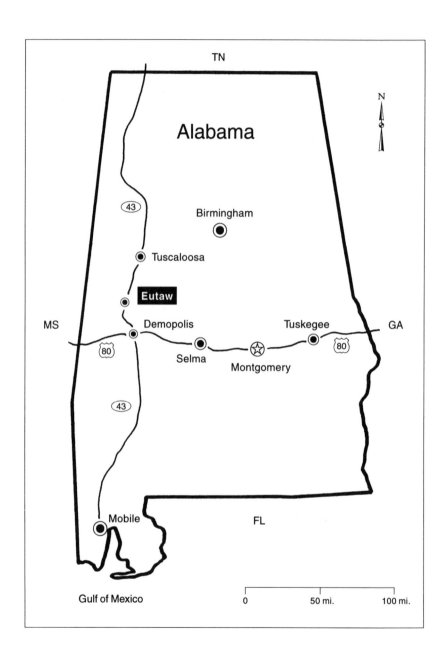

TN

Alabama

N

43

Birmingham
●

●  Tuscaloosa

●  **Eutaw**

MS

Demopolis                    Tuskegee              GA
●                                   ●
80                ●         ☆                80
          Selma    Montgomery

43

Mobile                          FL
●

Gulf of Mexico

0          50 mi.        100 mi.

# INTRODUCTION:

# GOING TO GREENE COUNTY

*Unraveling time in Eutaw,* Greene County, Alabama, demands seeing remnants of the past in just about everything.
A collective Deep South sense of the importance of engrav-
ing things in time is reflected in the everyday conversations
of Eutaw women who celebrate references to quilt making
and foot washing and find sanctity in flower gardening,
fresh squeezed lemonade, and hand-churned ice cream.

Most black people in Alabama center time in the movement for civil rights. Things there are defined as having happened either before or after that movement. In Greene
County, the majority of black folks born before and during
the movement—55 percent of Greene County's black population in 1967—were born at home with midwives. Even
though most of today's childbearing women go either to the
local community hospital or drive to the obstetrical center in
Tuscaloosa, doctors here know women who still want to
have their babies at home because they believe that "birthin'
ain't nothin' but natural."

Margaret Charles Smith, born in Greene County, Alabama, in 1906, is believed to be Alabama's oldest living midwife. With decades of experience behind her, Mrs. Smith
knows traditional home birthing like cooking chicken for

1

Sunday dinner. In the nearly 3,000 births she attended, she never lost a mother and rarely lost a baby. But in 1976 Alabama joined in the rush of southern states to pass laws ending the practices of lay midwives. Mrs. Smith attended her last birth at the age of seventy-five in 1981, five years after the law ended the issuance of new lay-midwife permits and allowed only nurse-midwives to be licensed. (Nurse-midwives, registered nurses with credentials from the American College of Nurse-Midwives, usually work in hospital settings.)

Between 1976 and 1981, over 150 black Alabama midwives lost their permits to practice. But lay midwifery's death encountered a mighty opposing force in Mrs. Smith. Although stripped of her practice, Mrs. Smith remained visible locally and nationally. She is the first black person to receive the keys to her hometown. She won honors at the first Black Women's Health Project Conference in Atlanta in 1983, and she later attended the Working Conference to Preserve Traditional Midwife Practices at Spelman College in Atlanta. Such recognition generated good feelings, but failed to restore her practice. Ten years ago, Mrs. Smith confessed to me in a rare moment of despair, "I never wanted plaques to hang on my wall. I wanted to be a midwife."

## Research and Audiotaping

Mrs. Smith believes that she is the first black woman in Greene County to be the focus of a book. Only recently have southern black women, particularly in rural areas, been able to find ways not just to tell their stories, but to participate in editing and publishing decisions about autobiographical material. The classic *Stars Fell on Alabama* presents a brief description of the mystical life of black prophetess Nancy Vaughn of Eutaw in the 1930s, and writers funded by the

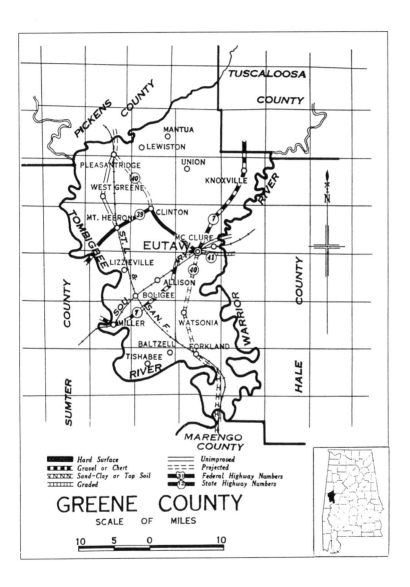

GREENE COUNTY

SCALE OF MILES

federal government during the Great Depression recorded slave narratives. Publication of *Motherwit*, the only other oral history of an Alabama midwife, apparently did not involve the storyteller as coauthor, although *Motherwit* was a groundbreaking book that received wide acclaim prior to the death in 1995 of Mrs. Onnie Lee Logan, a Mobile midwife.

I met Mrs. Smith in 1981 while I was documenting the experiences of Alabama's last generation of traditional midwives. When I left Alabama after interviewing sixty midwives, I kept in touch with several of them, including Mrs. Smith. Over the next thirteen years, I saw Mrs. Smith both at home and at such national lay-midwife meetings as the Midwife Alliance of North America (MANA) Conference in West Virginia and at The Farm in Tennessee. (The Farm is a spiritually based commune that has trained empirical midwives and vigorously supports home birth.) Some of my findings from these earlier interviews with Alabama midwives appear in this book.

In April 1992, over a catfish lunch, Mrs. Smith said, "I want a book about me." We immediately began planning for marathon tape-recording sessions and regular telephone conversations. From that moment until we completed the project in 1995, Mrs. Smith was a rigid taskmaster, ardent about meeting deadlines, setting goals, and staying on course.

The project resulted in many hours of new audiotaped interviews. We taped most often at her house, but sometimes in Atlanta or Birmingham. Early one morning I called on Mrs. Smith to tape before even getting out of bed—in a state between waking and dreaming. I also wrote down things she said to me just before she fell asleep at night. Some of the best interviews, however, occurred in the middle of the day in Mrs. Smith's living room, where the summer heat helped her to drift into a trance state ideal for allowing her recollections to roam freely. Our days of audiotaping sometimes ended with visits with her Eutaw friends and relatives—Mary Florence, Herlene Pipping, Laura Kate, Augusta Duncan, and others. These visits provided enjoyable breaks from our intense dialogues and offered opportunities for corroborating some of Mrs. Smith's experiences. Community letters solicited by Mrs. Smith and interviews with former clients of midwives and local doctors added to the scope of the research. Visits with Spiver Gordon, a long-time civil rights activist, "child of a midwife," and current Eutaw city councilman, provided additional information about civil and voting rights in Greene County.

I also made some use of a series of tape-recorded interviews with Margaret Charles Smith, April–November 1979, in the Archives of American Minority Culture, of the W. Stanley Hoole Special Collections at the University of Alabama. I have quoted portions of "Mama died at 101" with Mrs. Smith's permission. Readers can listen to tape recordings deposited at the Minority Archives and hear Mrs. Smith tell similar versions of some of the stories in this book.

## Editing

Mrs. Smith is a master at weaving words into memorable images. Her creativity adds much to the readability of the narrative. In recording her story, I was much more interested in preserving her way of speaking than in probing for exact times, dates, and places, but I have edited to give readers a more nearly linear account, although some flashbacks and examples of stream of consciousness remain.

Mrs. Smith was adamant about using the real names of friends and family members in the book. Ella Anderson, her midwife mentor, is one example. I believe that this is her way of recognizing people who remain nameless and voiceless in much of the literature. Mrs. Smith usually refers to doctors and nurses only by professional title, although Dr. Ruker Staggers is named in recognition of his support for her midwifery.

Each chapter opens with a brief historical description to give readers the proper context. In our conversations, I sometimes talked to Mrs. Smith about my other midwifery interviews or my own experiences, particularly in the area of reproductive health. During these times our work sessions were more like structured conversations than interviews. On occasion I sought information from other Eutaw residents, but they usually sent me back to Mrs. Smith as one of Greene County's most important repositories of Eutaw history.

In editing the transcripts, I was tempted to present Mrs. Smith in a way that would make her acceptable to present-day health care professionals. In a society where those who wield medical power tend to be members of the economic and social elite, I kept asking myself, what is the cost of failing to present Mrs. Smith in the image of today's health care professionals? Should I include traditions, or would they be misunderstood and labeled ignorant and backward? Some professional midwives have difficulty reconciling the image of the old-time southern black midwife with the formally trained professional nurse-midwife. In the end I realized that my task was simply to present her as she is.

She is a poet who flavors southern recitations that have standard amen corner–style responses with her own experiences. Such recitations usually chronicle never-ending economic hard times, the civil rights movement, and the Christian faith and can be heard in churches, on porches, or wherever black folks gather. But Mrs. Smith adds her midwifery experience. I listened carefully to how she related the experiences of being black, female, and a rural midwife.

Early on in the interviews, Mrs. Smith stitched together pieces of her life story, some involving the trials of sexual assault, pregnancy, childbirth, and hard work. Evidence of long-buried memories unfolded from death's winding sheets as she recalled her childhood in Greene County. I asked Mrs. Smith repeatedly about her wish to include the personal in the book, and she always responded that readers would be interested. Her self-perceptions were not blurred by any external biases of class, race, or gender.

In this book Mrs. Smith has allowed some of the anger that she usually leaves unexpressed to be recorded. Mrs. Smith is accomplished at moving in both black and white worlds. She has spent a lifetime assuming roles where she comforts, for example, white residents of Eutaw with reassuring words about "how time has moved just too fast." Some white Eutaw residents who read this book may be surprised by the hints of anger and the bluntness that sometimes characterize her tone. This voice contrasts sharply with the genteel spirit that she displays to the local white community at the bank or in the supermarket. In deciding to tell her story, Mrs. Smith has also decided to reveal her troubled spirit. She acknowledges her suffering and admits outrage at the treatment she received as a black woman and a midwife. Mrs. Smith does not expect everyone in Greene County to like this book. In fact, she has even joked, "After this book comes out, I may have to leave Greene County."

As we completed work on the book, I read several parts of the manuscript to Mrs. Smith as a way to edit the work collaboratively. I knew I was on target when I read the first part of a sentence and she finished it just as transcribed. Mrs. Smith's final recommendation for the book was that it be short enough to read on an average airplane ride. In August of 1995, she blessed the book by saying, "This book here is ready."

### *On Spiritual Ground*

The Rev. George Washington Carver, a prominent Montgomery minister whose grandmother was a midwife in Pickens County, once told me that the Bible could have been written by somebody going around talking to midwives. Perhaps this is because so many midwives credit their successes to their abilities to talk to God easily and readily, or perhaps it is because their stories illustrate how God works through them.

Mrs. Smith's spiritual sensibilities help her to face all the challenges of daily life. She usually expresses her devotion privately, and although she has been a lifelong member of the Rehobeth Primitive Baptist Church in Clinton (she also belongs to a lodge that collects fifty cents each month from members for burial fees), her midwifery called to her more strongly than churchgoing did. Today she religiously balances the negative with the positive; no matter how dark recollections of the past may be, she always pauses to recognize the spiritual significance of overcoming. For her, as for many black women in Alabama, such balancing is as basic as keeping one's word. Although she will enthusiastically point out blessings to anyone, she does not try to proselytize, but meets people at their spiritual level and supports them on their journey. When I was with Mrs. Smith, I entered a world where having the weather be right for taking pictures was a blessing from God, and where an ordinary bedroom was transformed into a heavenly resting place by her chanting the Christian mantra, "Thank you, Jesus. We just thank you, Jesus."

### *Place*

Winding down dusty dirt roads, seeing pine trees touch the sky, I opened myself to one of Alabama's transcendental experiences: hearing hums turn to moans like survival songs passed on from slave ships. I recall thinking that drops of rain were my own tears. Just seeing a sky cluttered with stars enraptured me, and witnessing the noonday sun transform a hillside into a stream of white, sparkling lights made nature a temple of thanksgiving.

It is often said that this region is a favored dwelling place for ghosts. People regularly tell stories of being born with the veil, or caul, over the face, which enables the person so born to see hants, wanton spirits, and other mysterious ramblings in setting moons and traveling lights. Places like Boligee, not far from Eutaw, where young boys gather in a vacant laundromat with broken windows, on a main street of nothingness, seem lost in time. Such places are remote in many ways from urban Atlanta and suburban Tuscaloosa.

Parts of Greene County, which covers approximately 637 square miles, are about twelve miles from Mississippi. Eutaw, the county seat, is only thirty-three miles from Tuscaloosa and about seventy-five from Birmingham. Greene County's population, according to 1990 U.S. Census data, is 10,153 persons; its black population accounts for 8,181 of them.

Today Greene County advertises itself as a haven of antebellum finds and welcomes tourists with interests in hunting, fishing, and visiting antebellum homes. A recent *New York Times* travel section article heralded Eutaw's charm and provided a guide for touring in Greene County. Digging for fossils is also a popular summer activity.

Signs of early habitation can be found in the mounds of the Choctaw Indian nations. In 1875, laborers building the Sardis Church not far from West Greene found a sacred burial ground. In digging, they unearthed twenty-five Native American bodies placed in a circle, with their heads pointing toward the center.

When I come into Eutaw, I immediately dive into the past. The town square has such familiar American markers as the A & P, Church's Chicken, coin-operated laundromats, video rental stores, and even a brand new county courthouse named after the first black to be elected probate judge, George McKinley Branch. But what I like about Eutaw is the old-fashioned dry-goods stores with wooden floors, overhead fans, and aging Coca-Cola murals. Raised from the street by a sidewalk with walk-up steps, the stores' extended tin roofs jut out over the sidewalk and protect shoppers from sun and rain.

Everyone in Eutaw can take advantage of the town square's set of hanging traffic lights to stare into passing cars. Experienced watchers don't need to look at license plates to identify newcomers. Relatives expecting guests get word from such watchers long before their visitors arrive.

Several middle-aged to elderly black men greet one's entry with solemn nods from their positions on milk crates outside the A & P. (I always need to get out at the A & P to use the pay phone to call Mrs. Smith for directions. I wonder if these men see my arrivals as the next episode of a soap opera, even though months go by between them.) They stare at me as if they've been there since stores provided what the farm couldn't, and the biggest event in black folks' life was coming to town on Saturday. Despite the political upheaval of the civil rights movement, many of the lost dreams of these middle-aged and older black men are the same as the unfulfilled hopes of the generations before them.

An occasional car blasting contemporary hip-hop music is a jarring reminder of my penchant for romanticism. For a moment, I thought there was no urban Top Ten here! Deep in the country, I have seen places where cows have taken over abandoned porches and rock on porch swings as if the Great Depression had never ended. But the rap sounds blaring from radios make it clear that this is the electronic age—and the back roads of Greene County have connections to New York. Suddenly I connect the old men's mumblings with rap pulsations. The geographical connections of black communities—North to South and back again—are ongoing. Many children and teenagers from cities like Detroit, Chicago, and New York spend their summers in Greene County.

### Marking Progress

While the Jim Crow signs are down, reminders of segregation remain in Eutaw's structures, attitudes, and habits. When Mrs. Smith rides through Eutaw, she describes the all-white high school, the houses built by slaves, and the old courthouse that used to be the slave market and the hanging place. Eutaw children who are descendants of slaves can point out the families who owned their great-grandmothers. A local doctor's office built in the 1960s still has the two waiting rooms that once separated white and black. The laws and the signs may be gone, but when I went to the doctor's office with Mrs. Smith, she pointed out how the races still self-segregate. She decided to sit on the white side.

Mrs. Smith remembers decades of having to walk through side and back doors when visiting white homes. Recently we were warmly received at a local white doctor's home. Memories resurfaced from the beginning of this encounter, however, as Mrs. Smith reflected on which door to use when entering. After some discussion, she chose to ring the side doorbell.

The past also lingers in the behavior of a prominent white family's elementary school child. With affection that stems from years of Mrs. Smith's caretaking, he enthusiastically greets Mrs. Smith as "Margaret." Older blacks still cringe when they recall demeaning references to them as

11

"boy" or "girl" coupled with mandates for them always to refer to whites by title and surname.

When addressing how midwives were cut off from practice in Alabama after the civil rights movement, Mrs. Smith is as thoughtful and analytical as she is when looking at how far black people have come since civil rights. She refuses to be locked into relating folk stories about past birthing experiences. Her voice rises like that of a Baptist minister taking a sermon to its height when describing midwifery achievements. She demands me to be "listening good" when she talks about how white doctors just didn't care about poor black women. When comparing past home births with contemporary hospital births, Mrs. Smith is militant in her criticism of doctors who are too busy to spend time with women. Mrs. Smith reminds her audiences that midwives stayed with women for as long as they were needed.

### Back to Midwifery

Mrs. Smith remains a giant presence in her small town. She stands like a tree refusing to be felled in a field cleared for pasture. Although she walks with shoulders slightly stooped, perhaps from years of bending to pick cotton, she is a woman of enormous physical strength. In the middle of her full-moon face are deepset owl eyes framed by charcoal eyebrows with no hint of gray. Life's hardships have not clouded her forehead. Mrs. Smith stands over six feet tall, and her bearing is always royal, no matter what she happens to be wearing. She used to wear straw hats—she never leaves home with her head uncovered—but now she usually wears store-bought turban-style caps. Because of swelling in her feet, Mrs. Smith slips on her black Reeboks for comfort more times than she would like when going to town. (Like many Alabama women, when she is at home or in the yard, she prefers to go barefoot.) But no matter how casual her town mission may be, she always wears a dress, never pants.

The conversations Mrs. Smith has with people when she goes into Eutaw include asking about family members, talking about babies she has delivered, and finding out who might be pregnant now. Young women in their twenties come up to Mrs. Smith and ask to hear the stories of their own births. Among these stories are accounts of women who would pull up in labor in Mrs. Smith's yard just a few years ago. Their excuse? They got lost on the way to the hospital—the hospital that's in the opposite direction.

Mrs. Smith continues her midwifery by giving advice. One woman is anticipating her daughter's giving birth. She asks Mrs. Smith, "Should she go now or wait for the due date to come?" Only when she has used her powers of discernment to determine what the mother really wants to do will Mrs. Smith reply, "If you can go, go as soon as you can." Another Eutaw resident asks Mrs. Smith about a niece whose doctor said she might have trouble giving birth. Then there is the young pregnant girl whose mother is in jail. Mrs. Smith visits her in Eutaw's low-rent housing projects. Holding her hand and rubbing her back, she offers comfort, telling her having that baby won't be as hard as she thinks. Mrs. Smith keeps her door open to anyone seeking support. She can dig into hearts and read minds to find what is hurting and heal it.

Just a generation ago, midwives attended most Alabama women. Young adults in Eutaw still shout, "Mrs. Smith delivered me!" Across the South, people say, "I'm a midwife's child!" Or they'll explain the importance of midwives by saying simply, "They got us here." As Mary Florence of Eutaw explained, "When I got in labor, I thought I was supposed to have Margaret Smith."

Waiting for a midwife revival in Greene County is easy. Calendars don't always change with the years. Hands on

*Introduction*

clocks often stand still. Midwife spirits are passing by
constantly. A world is born every time a Greene County
storyteller begins, "Before and after the movement, we
had midwives." Surely time will come again for midwifery
in Alabama: Midwives like Mrs. Smith specialize in waiting
on time.

*Just don't tell them all you know.* That's one thing you don't do. You tell them what you want them to know, and what you don't want them to know, don't tell them. You got to use common sense here, because we got a long ways—like a long ways—still to go.

—Margaret Charles Smith

# | 1 |

# GROWING UP

*Slavery was just moments away.* In the early twentieth century, women who had survived the auction block, involuntary separation from their families, and cruel sexual molestation cared for children and grandchildren born after emancipation. Some shared their accounts of surviving the whip; others chose to spare the next generation the most heinous details of slavery. In grim references to what they called the "dark days," midwives told me what their grandmothers had told them—about eating from pig troughs, praying into tin tubs filled with water to mute the sound, using mandated passes for travel, and being raped by white men. Mrs. Smith learned much about the past from her grandmother, and she too experienced deep suffering and discontent when coming of age in Greene County.

## Greene County in Slavery and in Freedom

As one of Alabama's wealthiest plantation regions, Greene County was unequivocally a land of slavery. Many of its first settlers journeyed westward from South Carolina with slaves in tow. Between 1820 and 1840 the population of Greene County swelled from 4,554 to 24,024. Nearly four-fifths of the inhabitants were slaves. The county's population peaked in 1860 at 30,859 inhabitants. This belt of land, called the Black Belt, was known for its rich black soil, kept fertile

17

by Greene County's rivers—the Sipsey, the Black Warrior, and the Tombigbee—as well as by countless streams and creeks. In Greene County's golden era, slave labor and fertile soil made cotton king.

To control the large slave population, the Deep South states passed and adhered to a harsh slave code. In 1852 Alabama slaves were legally stripped of all basic rights, including freedom to own property, seek work, gather together, make speeches, keep or carry a gun, and even freedom of movement. Another Alabama law, which remained on the books until after the Civil War, made teaching slaves to read and write punishable by imprisonment, fines, or both. Female slaves were, in addition, subjected to sexual abuse and medical experimentation. Between 1845 and 1849 J. Marion Sims, a pioneer American gynecologist who developed the speculum, conducted a series of vaginal surgeries on Alabama slave women. White women found the pain from the procedure intolerable, but several black slaves were forced to endure dehumanizing operations repeatedly without anesthesia. Although medical knowledge and use of anesthesia were limited at the time, at least one major medical journal reported the effectiveness of nitrous oxide and inhaled ether as an anesthetic as early as 1846, according to a scholarly article in *Sage*, a black women's academic journal.

On February 11, 1865, less than a year before the Thirteenth Amendment to the Constitution officially ended slavery, S. S. Brown, who lived in Greene County, wrote to Mr. Foster Kirksey, a prominent Eutaw landowner and former Greene County sheriff, to complain about a slave's apparent effort to reunite with her husband. Brown wrote: "The negro woman Ann that I hired went home after her clothes and has not returned. She went 2 weeks ago today without my permission. I think she went to your Boligee place. I do not wish to be bothered with her, and she having a husband on your place & you seem to want her, if you will take her, I will pay you for the time I have had her in possession." In Greene County, blacks risked severe whippings and other forms of violent punishment for going anywhere without a pass.

During Reconstruction, blacks in Greene County and elsewhere experienced new freedoms. As former slaves pushed for their rights—to vote, to make money, to move to town—they met growing and sometimes violent resistance. Eutaw was considered an oasis of culture by some, with its two newspapers, its bookstore, its learning academies for males and females, and its Greek Revival architecture. But it was also a hot spot for white terrorism, Ku Klux Klan organizing, and lawlessness.

In 1867 local white residents burned down the courthouse to destroy what they viewed as damaging Reconstruction records. White violence broke out again three years later when a crowd numbering approximately eighteen hundred to two thousand blacks gathered at the courthouse to support a progressive political slate of candidates. About two hundred conservative white Democrats stood on the sidelines and shot into the crowd, killing two and injuring an estimated thirty, according to local newspaper reports.

In the short-lived Reconstruction years, families struggled to hold on to their meager economic gains. In 1875, Henry Charles, Mrs. Smith's grandmother's husband, filed a deed at the Greene County courthouse. He bequeathed his wife several items of personal property, including two mules and several cows. It was hard enough for blacks just out of slavery to achieve self-sufficiency with Reconstruction laws promoting equity among the races; when Jim Crow became the law of the land, their dreams turned into nightmares. The Jim Crow laws passed after Reconstruction legalized a kind of apartheid. The Supreme Court's ruling in *Plessy v. Ferguson* (1896) permitted "separate but equal" facilities for blacks and whites—never a reality—and opened the way to legal segregation on trains and buses, in housing and working conditions, restaurants, theaters, hospitals, playgrounds, and all other public recreational areas. Simultaneously, poll taxes, literacy tests, and violence disfranchised blacks who had voted after the Civil War. And the practice of sharecropping and other more independent forms of agricultural labor left blacks struggling economically, experiencing a reenslavement without chains.

## *Alabama Medicine*

When Booker T. Washington arrived in Alabama from the Hampton Institute in 1881, he found no licensed black physicians, pharmacists, or dentists. In the mid-1880s a black man, Cornelius Nathaniel Dorsett, passed the six-day Alabama medical examination. Dr. Dorsett later helped form the National Medical Association, the professional association for black doctors. In 1891, Dr. Halle Tanner Dillon Johnson became the first woman ever to be licensed by the Alabama Medical Society. A black woman and an early graduate of Philadelphia's Woman's Medical College, Dr. Johnson found overwhelming medical need in the Black Belt of Alabama. Booker T. Washington recruited Johnson to come to the Tuskegee Institute. While she was there, Johnson sought funds to build a dispensary. In comments prepared in 1894 for the Nineteenth Annual Meeting of the Alumnae Association of the Woman's Medical College of Pennsylvania, Johnson reported that families living far from town could not afford medical care because physicians charged two dollars per mile for a visit—plus the cost of medicine—and demanded cash or reliable assurances of payment before coming. Dr. Johnson also described the widespread poverty of the region: "In the vicinity of our school are hundreds in need

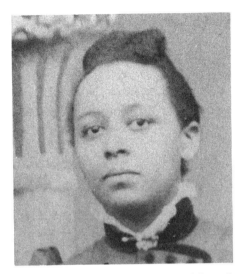

Dr. Halle Tanner Dillon Johnson, Alabama's first licensed female doctor, 1891. Archives and Special Collections on Women in Medicine, Medical College of Pennsylvania and Hahnemann University (MCPHU).

of medical attention. Children with tubercular tendencies, sore eyes, various skin troubles, and in a pitiable condition generally. Women with faces bearing the marks of pain upon them; faces which testify but too plainly that life is a burden with such diseased bodies" (106–7). In her conclusion, she testified to the strength of the black population, even those in dire poverty. "If you could see how often, in spite of adverse circumstances, they pull through and get well, it would put in doubt the much-advanced theory that colored persons are readier to succumb to disease than whites. With all that they have to contend with, I wonder that any of them live" (ibid.).

For health care, most black women in Greene County relied on each other and on an array of indigenous healers and folk practitioners, including midwives. They established a system of mutual aid and self-help. Cooperation and assistance grew out of kinship, neighborhood, church, and family ties. From slavery on, black women had provided birthing care to women white and black, earning respect in both communities. From the beginning of public health regulation, some doctors were hostile to midwives, unwilling to recognize them as appropriate caregivers. H. Y. Webb, a frustrated Greene County health officer, wrote on May 25, 1889, "Every Negro woman who has had one or two children thinks herself perfectly competent to discharge all the duties of a Midwife." Even when the midwives were more experienced, bias against them was the norm. Categorizing blacks generally in pejorative terms, the health officer complained in a letter to the state health officer on October 18, 1882, "The Negroes are ignorant—& there are 18166 of them—My own beat and Town are all right—Some of the Beats have no Doctors living in them—I have only been enabled to get the names of about 20 Midwives in the County. These are the Regulars—They are a prolific race commence bearing children at 12 years . . . irregular midwives are counted by the hundred" (Alabama Department of Health, State Health Officer's correspondence). A Knoxville, Alabama, gynecologist, Dr. Thomas W. Pierce, was more paternalistic in his assessments of the midwife situation in Greene County: "As to the midwives, about every other Negro woman is a midwife, and frequently the parturient waits upon herself—but I am satisfied if the doctors took sufficient interest in the matter, there would be no difficulty in getting them all to report, for the negro as a tendency is very pliable and can be led to do any thing, especially where they feel there is honor attached to it. I keep a list of a few important midwives when I can ascertain [their] whereabouts." In one town the schoolteacher even listed a local midwife's births, providing a community service.

The frustration and hostility of the white medical establishment toward black midwives stands in sharp contrast to the respect these women earned in their own communities. White doctors ignored the problems midwives faced in aiding neighbors struggling in poverty and oppressed by the social, political, and economic conditions of the Jim Crow South. Throughout her youth, Mrs. Smith witnessed hard times and endured strict disciplinary measures. She spent most of her childhood working. She says, "We worked our ass off all through the week and we had no money and no clothes to show for it." But she also remembers the strength of women in her community with pride: "People cared about each other back then."

---

I WAS RAISED BY A SLAVERY TIME LADY. That's who raised me. She was brought to this country and sold, put on a stage and sold for three dollars, her and three more. I always heard Mama say she could near about name the people that were brought to this country with her. They brought Margaret Smith, Miss Lucy Cockrell, and one other lady. Miss Lucy Cockrell is dead and gone, and all of her sisters are dead and gone. But some of her children are still living. We were all raised up together. They all used to stay on the other side of the hard road. They called it "off 14." And all of us used to be on the old road, Calhoun Road, that was when it was a dirt road, blacktop now. My grandmother who raised me was brought in by some white people they called the Charleses, and that's why we went with Charles. They had to give them a name because they didn't have one. They were put up on a stage, just like you auction something, right down where the courthouse

23

is now. My grandmother said she was about thirteen turning fourteen when they brought them here. See, her name was Margaret. They named me after her. Those white people who bought her named her.

She stayed with the same white people the entire time. She came here and was raised and worked as a slave for them in their house until she got big enough or old enough to marry. When we got ready to go somewhere, I remember her telling me that she wasn't allowed to go nowhere unless she had a pass. They had a certain time to go and a certain time to be back. They used to wouldn't allow them to go nowhere. And they had a certain man they had to marry when they got ready to marry because he had to be a breeding man. They couldn't go with just anything. He had to be a man that could bring forth fruit.

When the freedom come, white folks didn't tell them they were free. They kept on working like slaves. The Yankees had to tell it. The white folks wouldn't want me telling this now, but it's true.

See, my grandmother who raised me, her husband's name was Henry, Henry Charles. Henry left his wife a lifetime home. There used to be some great big old oak trees over there. Her husband brought them out the swamp with switches, I'm talking about. They make log cabins now, but not like they used to make them. They built a log house and the log was hewed on both sides, just right smooth with a chop ax. That's what we were born and raised in. Once the roof got to leaking, had to throw a tin roof on top. But that's the only thing we put on to the house. It was all wood. Wooden windows—threw them open. Wooden doors—threw them open. Even had wooden pins holding the logs together. That house was hard to tear down.

24

My grandmother told me often, they worked for that land, slavery. They didn't pay but fifty cents an acre, and they got it. They saved it, I imagine, by eating scarce and doing without things. We hauled wood to town, taking it to different white people because they had chimneys in that day, you know, wood was the style. And I reckon that is the way they saved a little money. And she was still working for white people right on, but she wasn't getting nothing.

It was hard for you to get land, but I reckon they were thinking that this was swamp, just like over there was swamp, we would call it. They would get a gallon of whiskey and cook what they had and have logrollings. They would tell the people to come and help them to roll logs, burn logs and things like that, clean it up. Men would roll the logs and make a big fire and burn the logs up and all the brush. Then they have dinner for them. She said that they had to clean up every stitch of that land when they got it, work. Her husband would get this gallon of whiskey for people who drank whiskey. They just have a big time on Saturday. That was their day. They would clean up so much today, and probably what they could during the week. When they weren't in the field, they would do a whole lot.

Just like they got this place cleaned up, then they go on to another place. Just like when we were growing up, when we got through chopping cotton this week, next week we had to go over there and help those people finish. That's the way we had to do. That's the way it used to be, but there ain't no more days like that now.

Just like if somebody got sick, the house would be full that evening by sundown. People would sit all night long, but they don't do that no more. They sit right there till they die, get better, or one. There be a group coming tonight and a group

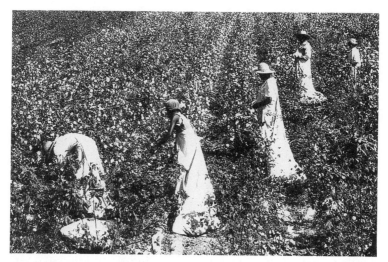

Women picking cotton in the 1920s. National Archives, Records of the Office of the Secretary of Agriculture.

coming another night, but that t'ain't no more. If somebody was sick, they would come, you know, in droves. I don't hear tell of it no more, nowhere I go, nowhere.

Now my grandmother's mama was sick. And people would be coming, riding horses and mules, walking, and I was real small, but I didn't know really what was going on. But they was coming to sit with her that night. If she needed anything or if she happened to pass, they would be there. So that's the way that was. Four or five women come tonight. Four or five women come tomorrow night.

Some come daytime and wash, iron, scrub, do anything, clean the house up, stay all night. Then tomorrow the next group come in, wash and scrub, put on peas and greens, whatever, and then they go. If somebody was lying up in front of death, if she needed anything, they would be there.

## Motherless Child

I was supposed to be named under Sanders. That was my mother's name, Beulah Sanders. My mother gave me to my grandmother, the lady who raised me. I just loved her to death, but she was rough. She worked you now. You wasn't going to sit down. See, some people were in tight places. They had so many children. And they couldn't provide for them. She raised ten of us in her lifetime and weren't any of them her own. All the others were grown when I come along. I was the last one, me and Dennis.

I had no mother. I don't know who my daddy was or nothing. That's the worse part. I never did ask, and they never sat down and really told me things. You couldn't say things to old people, like children say to old people now, 'cause you got your tail tore up.

They just didn't talk in front of children because there were some things that they weren't supposed to know. She used to bring it up on occasion about what my mother told her just before she died. My mama told my grandmother that she wanted her to raise me.

She just told me, "Now, you are getting to be a big girl. Your mother passed when you were three weeks old, so they say. You were the only child your mother had."

I said, "Yes'm."

She said, "Your mama told me to whoop you and raise you so everyone would care for you."

I said, "Yes'm."

But I said to myself, "You already got blisters on my butt now."

I asked my grandmother who raised me, "What happened?"

She said, "I had to go to field and I left her at the house, and

27

I don't know what she ate or what she drank while I was away."

But Lucy, she's the one who told it. Lucy used to cornbraid my hair. She's the one who told me my mama got out the bed and went to the pear tree and got a bucket of pears and came back and ate every one of them and died, died that night.

## Lots of Work and Little Schooling

I tell you, children these days don't know nothing about work. I had to fall in that swamp every evening to get them cows out of there and bring them to the house. And better not be till dark getting them neither. They had nine head of cows. I better get on where they were. They had on bells. You stop and listen for the bells. You could tell what direction they were in, up thataway, down thataway, or 'cross yonder.

I called grandmother my mama, and she went to making Dennis go get the cows and pen them. She also made Dennis cut the wood, and I'd tote it. Like if the weather is going to be bad, if she saw a drove of geese coming in, she'd tell us, "Well, you all got to tote wood tomorrow. It's going to be bad weather, and you wanna get it up before it gets bad." And sure enough, the next day or two, it get cold and rainy.

Dennis didn't like that toting wood so well. But did she whoop! She really whooped. Dennis said that he was getting to be a big boy now. He was a man. But when Mama got through whipping his tail, I'm telling you the truth, he wished he was a child. She'd burn you up.

She always tell you, "I can't afford to buy you clothes, I'll have to make your dress." We had dresses made with buttons down the back and a belt to go around and a big button back there. I tore mine off. I never did like buttons, and I'd get a killing about my dress. We had a calico for Christmas. You don't see that material now, had some sort of red in it. I was about fifteen years old before I had my first pair of shoes, slippers. We went barefoot most of the year, but I did get those old hard brogan shoes, laced up in the front, what we wore to school. They were so hard that you couldn't bend them. Better not wear them out. You weren't going to get no more. That's the truth. Then I got some baby-doll patent leathers that you greased with tallow to make them shine. We had the shoes called baby dolls. I was a happy soul. I wore them to church and then pulled them off soon as I got home. Got me a rag and brushed them off real good, and put them up.

The last time Mama whooped me, I bit her. The old folks had a knack of putting your head in between your legs and twisting that coattail like this here. And, boy that fair bootie be out there, oooh! Dennis would fool me into things and then he back up. He said he didn't do it. I did it. Make both of us get a whooping.

I was big enough to kill chickens and cook them. Sometimes Dennis gave me the wing. Sometimes he gave me the drumstick. Sometimes he wouldn't give me that.

There were some colored people that had a bigger family and had more opportunity to work and do than my mama did 'cause Mama was getting old, and she couldn't do what she wanted to do. We just had to take what we could get and go along with it, but she fed us. Cooked on a fireplace, made biscuits, and put them in the skillet. You couldn't tell them from those that come out of a stove. You got that cornbread with those peas and greens, every day, every day. Lord, turnips every day.

Bless your soul, we had to, me and Dennis, had to sweep that yard before we went to school. We had to get that dirt from under the house. We had to sweep that trash out from under there from where the chickens were. Better not leave anything under there, for we could get a killing and go to school hurting.

School was open for three months, 'cause we come out in February. We had to get on them ditch banks and clean them ditch banks off. Just like a ditch run down through here and have briars and bushes on in it. You had to take a hoe and clean that ditch bank off. That's before you started plowing. Then, after we did that, we had to get a stick and get out there and knock them cotton stalks backwards and forth, backwards and forth. Children today don't know half of what I know. I didn't get much of a chance to go to school. We had to stop and go to field.

To get to that school, you have to go straight up that road for about a mile and a half, then turn off this road and go down through the swamp and come out of it in a pasture. And get out the pasture and go up the hill to the Smith School. It was over in Pine Grove. There was lots of colored living there. The road was full of us going to school. They called it Smith's place over in the sixteenth section. The people donated the pine logs, and the plantation owner permitted them to build a school. It was one big room and had a shed back there to put the wood in. I never would forget that. Toting all that wood. I be worn out toting the wood at home before we got there. When we got to school, we had to tote wood to make a fire. That's what killed me. Boys would go out there and cut the wood, and girls tote it. We tote it up. Plenty of boys up there to cut enough wood to tote it tomorrow.

That teacher was a colored teacher. That's all we had back then, colored school and a colored teacher. She whooped you, so help me. Look like she just beat you till there wouldn't be a hand. She was humped. She had a knot in her back. Her head was carried down. She was as mean as she wanted to be. Anybody could tell anything about you, and she believed them.

I told Mama one evening when I came home, "I can't use my right hand."

She said, "What ails your hand?"

I said, "My teacher hit it off near 'bout."

Mama said, "Well, if it didn't drop off, she didn't do nothing."


## Trapped in Greene County

Dennis promised me that whenever he left he would come back and get me. He promised me so faithful that the next time Mama whooped him he was going to go. He said, "I'm too big for her to whoop me."

But she ate his tail up. I wasn't old enough to amount to nothing. I reckon I was about twelve going on thirteen.

Dennis was 'bout up in his teens somewhere, something like eighteen or nineteen when he left. And he promised me that he would come back to get me just as soon as he found him some work to do.

I didn't ask him any questions about where he was going to live. I didn't have sense enough, I reckon. I was just looking for him to come back and say, "Let's go."

I was ready to go. I was going to slip off. Do something. I was going to get away from here. I just looked and looked and looked and looked and looked. The Lord fixed it where he didn't come back.

When I saw Dennis again, he had his jawbone ripped up. A saw ripped his gum and teeth, and his mouth was kind of twisted. He was working at a sawmill. You hardly knew him.

I said to myself, "I'd be so glad when I get grown, I don't know what to do."

But when you're grown, you wish you were back to being a child.

## *Seeing Flowers*

I wanted a sister so bad. I'd get me a stick just juggling, trying to find me a baby. They used to say those babies come out the stump. I looked in every stump and ain't seen none yet. Late getting the cows in 'cause I wanted me a sister. They said you get them out the stump with a stick, juggling.

I told Mama, "I thought you always said babies come in stumps."

I looked in every stump and ain't seen none yet. Once a courting girl had a baby, they didn't allow us to associate, she done had a baby. She done wrong. You couldn't sit aside her. You couldn't play with her. But I'm so fast, I'm going up there to see her. I wanted to see that baby, but I was scared to go. Old folks call Mama before I got there 'cause she got a baby. You ask somebody how you got a baby, you might get a killing. You run your mouth too much, your tail got tore up.

But Sam Duncan, we used to walk to school together. He was out there dating women. I asked him and at first he wouldn't tell it 'cause he said you get a killing. Then he told it. He said, "Margaret, kissing don't get it. A girl that done laid down and a man laid on top of her, that girl let a man get between her legs."

See, folks had been saying I was good. My mama did tell me, "Now you seen your flowers, that's what they called your period, you're old enough to get a baby. Don't let ne'er a boy touch you, 'cause you might come up with a baby." And that's all she said. But kissing don't get it. A girl's got to lie down.

They used to give you an old piece of quilt to make your

pad and tie a string around your waist. But I didn't know what was happening. I reckon I was fixing to die. I slept in the bed right there beside Mama, and I saw that blood. I thought she was going to whip me, but she didn't whip me.

She just told me, "Margaret, you've seen your flowers. You are a young lady."

## Old-Time Religion

I always told my mama that I wanted to be where she was. Everyone was together then, but they've split apart now. See, the Primitive Baptist people split up. I stayed with Old Rehobeth Primitive Baptist Church. I helped build that church. That's Mama's church, belonged to it sixty-seven-odd years before she passed. That was an old church. I'd say we have a good forty, forty-five members. But one group went this way and that group went thataway. The big difference between the Primitive and the Baptists is that the Baptists don't wash feet and the Primitive do. Every September, they start the first Sunday, going to different churches around. Now there won't be any more foot washing till May. Come back in May. Wash feet twice a year unless a broke-down member somewhere hasn't had his feet washed in a good while by the members. A group of them will go that Sunday and wash So-and-So's feet. Everyone dressed in white, robes tied around, and head covered with white.

But back then, folks used to be terrible. They have foot washing, and those were the big days. Folks be in the woods drinking whiskey, shooting, and carrying on. One time I had to run till I broke my shoe heel off. They were shooting down through the crowd and, great goodness, shooting at a woman.

The foot washing was on, and just like you on recess, and

you come out till they turn the benches. See, they turn the benches. When you wash my feet, I turn around and wash your feet. That yard was just full of folks when that man commenced to shooting. I tore up them little six-dollar slippers, running. That heel just popped right on off. I must have hit a root or something. I had to work, scuffle, put back till I could get me some more shoes. I said look a-here, ain't got no money to get no more.

Listen to me good now, when the Lord frees your soul, you can't hold it. You got to get out, if you don't do any more than talk to the bushes and the posts and things. You don't have a private religion when the Lord frees your soul. You have been forgiven for your sins. He gives you a clean heart. Some folks go to church right today to see how can I outdress you. See So-and-So, and wasn't that dress a mess she had on. Well, that ain't no way. You supposed to let your heart go out for the person that doesn't have it. If you could, talk to some more people. Let's do so-and-so for So-and-So. That's what God wants. He loves his children. But some folks go to church just to see if they can outdress you. They work hard and get some fine clothes and just to go to church and twist, just twist. I just want to be clean and decent. I don't want to be looking like I come out the cotton patch. That's what God wants. Dress, He don't want it. Finery, He don't want it. He wants the pure in heart. Shall see God. That's right. That's right.

# | 2 |

# PREGNANCY

*In the tenant-farm system,* women had few choices about anything. When it came time for birth, who delivered their babies and where the babies were born had much more to do with rural isolation, race, and economics than with choice. Some women told me that they just managed to get to their cabins from the cotton fields in time to make a pallet on the floor to catch their own infants. Sometimes close family members and friends provided emotional support before and after the birth. Even when a community midwife or a doctor who might be hired by the plantation owner was called, the baby might be born before the official birth attendant arrived. On some occasions, however, women like Mrs. Smith wanted or had to guide themselves through the birthing process, seeking help only to cut and tie the umbilical cord.

Under Jim Crow law, most white hospitals remained segregated, and white nurses were instructed not to touch black male patients. A patchwork of mostly small hospitals provided some medical care for blacks in Birmingham, Montgomery, Selma, and Tuskegee. Women in Greene County seldom used such facilities because they were unfamiliar, far away, and costlier than midwife care. These early black hospitals, which had only a small number of beds, sometimes lay empty as a result of distrust about hospital care. Dr. John A. Kenney, the first medical director of

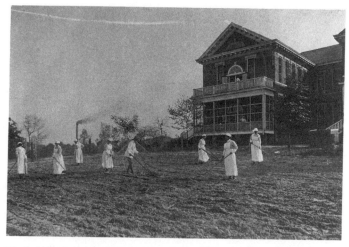

Nurses working on lawn at the Tuskegee Institute, 1912. Tuskegee University, Hollis Burke Frissell Library.

Tuskegee's John A. Andrew Memorial Hospital, wrote in *Services of a Negro Hospital:*

> It has been no simple task in this section to induce people to come to the hospital for treatment, because, isolated as they are, they have inherited the very common and very erroneous idea that a hospital is the last resort in case of sickness. It has required patience, perseverance and education gradually to change this idea. It was rather difficult to make the Tuskegee students feel at home in the hospital, and the admission of an outside patient from the surrounding communities was a rarity. (3)

The massive exodus of blacks to the North in the late 1920s brought some black women to urban hospital maternity wards for the first time. But for Greene County's remaining 16,263 blacks, who lived in the throes of economic depression (according to 1930 U.S. Census data), home birth with midwives remained the most common way of birth. Large tracts of the most productive land remained in the hands of a few of Greene County's 3,482 whites, and the wives of Eutaw's economic elite used doctors for their home births. As blacks elsewhere claimed a new voice in the Harlem Renaissance and the emerging Pan-African movements, Greene County blacks remained locked in an agricultural system that ensured their political silence. The ravages of the boll weevil reduced the cotton yield. Rapid soil deterioration and a lack of crop diversity further added to economic woes. Although after slavery ended blacks in Greene County joined an ill-fated attempt to establish a colony in Mexico, signs of black empowerment seemed to have been left behind in the nineteenth century.

Money was seldom exchanged, and blacks remained dependent on the plantation owner's system of bookkeeping, which determined how medical care, food, and other supplies would be doled out. County probate judges could place liens on crops, livestock, or anything else a family might own. The plantation way of life, with its exploitation of laborers, seemed much like slavery.

## Medicinal Plants in Greene County

In 1930, Greene County had no county health unit or any other system providing prenatal care. Occasionally women gave themselves some such special attention as rubbing their abdomens with castor oil, lard, or whatever lubricant might be on hand. Some of the older Alabama midwives used their skills in massage to position babies for birth. When labor began, many women remained active with domestic or farm work. This regular and sustained activity may have contributed to healthy birth outcomes.

It is not surprising that women often depended on their own gardens and the woods for their birthing pharmacopoeia.

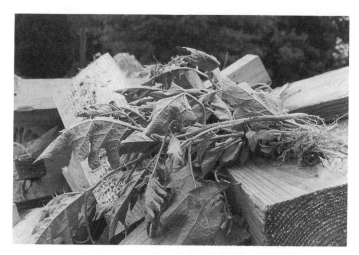

Eutaw tread sash. Photo by Linda Janet Holmes.

While common names for some indigenous plants varied across the state, the midwives I interviewed commonly reported using the following substances to induce labor: black haw, black pepper, mayapple root, ginger root, dirt dauber or spiderwebs, and tread sash tea. Tread sash has a prickly green leaf and grows freely in the Eutaw area.

The reasons for using a particular root or substance were sometimes forgotten or were kept secret to avoid ridicule. Knowing the concentration of a plant used for medicine, its dosage, and how to prepare it for administration sometimes determined whether a particular herb acted as a toxin or a medicine. References to several of these medicinal plants can be found in herbal literature. Some midwives agreed that such substances as black pepper, tread sash, ginger, and bamboo briar provoked the desired bodily heat and perspiration for activating contractions. Others, for example, dirt dauber tea, appeared to work by encouraging vomiting. Black pepper could cause sneezing and stimulate contractions. Along with teas and massage during labor, some midwives kept mothers hot by putting hot towels on the abdomen or by giving hot baths in the early stages of labor. The bamboo briar root, which has over twenty different species, is recognized for assisting in expelling the placenta and was used to hasten labor, but we do not know which species was used by Greene County midwives. Such herbs as hot ginger also helped bring on overdue menstruation.

Spirits of turpentine, camphor, quinine, and castor oil had multiple uses among both the white and the black rural populations. Sweet gum, mullein leaf, catnip, and horehound are age-old remedies whose multiple uses include bringing down fevers in children and curing cold symptoms. Jimsonweed was also used for reducing fevers. In 1931, Dr. Clarence K. Weil wrote to Peter Brannon, director of the Alabama archives, about the use of "Jamestown weed," which is believed to be the same as jimsonweed. Dr. Weil, in his description for the Brannon Collection of numerous practices current among local blacks, wrote, "The leaves of the Jamestown weed are salted and bound to the forehead to relieve fever." He added, "Canna leaves are used for the same purpose. Asafetida bag is supposed to relieve colic and many other infectious diseases" (Weil to Brannon, July 2, 1931).

Other remedies include castor oil, which has been known to intensify labor at least from the time of the Egyptians. The Egyptians also used honey to help the womb heal. Sugar has commonly been used for this purpose, and recent medical research has corroborated the usefulness of granulated sugar and povidone-iodine for accelerating womb healing.

While doctors may have scorned midwives' remedies, some white communities welcomed black midwives in spite of prevailing racial prejudices. A. L. Tommie Bass, a self described "old-timer herbist" living in Cherokee County,

Alabama, remembers one black midwife's medicines being used by white men and women in his community. While some southern accounts use references to voodoo to deride midwifery practices, the following quotation makes note of a midwife's skill in removing curses—not to be confused with a root doctor's ability to place one. He recalled in *Herbal Medicine Past and Present*: "We didn't have a big time herbist. People got their own herbs from the field or the store. There was Aunt Molly Kirby, they called her, a great big black woman. She made herb medicines and hoodoos. Lots of men went to her when they had social diseases. She was also a midwife, delivered worlds of babies. She'd go out on the mountain and deliver babies. They didn't allow colored people out there much, but they'd allow her" (39).

## *Worldwide Cultural Traditions*

Their connection to their ancestral roots meant that some older black Alabama midwives never relegated their practices to superstition or abandoned them. Practices that paralleled West African traditions included: abdominal massage and palpation during pregnancy; beliefs in marking babies with prenatal impressions; soups highly seasoned with pepper to encourage uterine contractions; medicinal baths at the onset of labor; maintaining a birth fire into the postpartum period; burial of the placenta near a tree; placing a sharp knife under the birthing bed or baby's bed (also practiced by white women in Appalachian regions); giving the baby an oil bath right after birth; naming the baby on the seventh or ninth day because its spirit is unsettled before then; and guarding against future use of the placenta by medicine men or others who wished to harm the mother.

Descriptions of birthing positions recommended by many women, including Mrs. Smith, parallel obstetrical field notes from parts of the world as far apart as West Africa and Southeast Asia. Sanya Dojo Onabamiro observed that in parts of Nigeria, at the time of confinement, a woman's husband called the medicine man and two or three elder women from the community. Children were asked to leave the house, and an inner room was swept clean to prepare for the labor and birth.

> When eventually the membranes rupture and the birth of the child is deemed to be nigh, the inmates of the room immediately take action stations. Two cushions are placed on the floor which has been previously covered with some medicinal mats, and the woman, now completely stripped, is asked to kneel down on those two cushions, knees far apart. The old woman sits behind her on a high stool and holds her up by clasping her under the arms. The woman is now urged to take deep breaths and make forceful bearing down efforts. (28)

Heat, universally associated with healing and relaxation, was encouraged in the birthing environment. Several Alabama women I interviewed described the fire in the mother's room as a special birth fire. No fire could be taken from it, and ashes in the fireplace could not be removed from the house, which sometimes resulted in overflowing buckets of ashes in the mother's room. Some West African cultures have similar birth fires.

Southern black midwifery shows parallels with other cultures in the customs surrounding the burial of the afterbirth. In Alabama, special measures for burial of the afterbirth, "the life of the mother," required salting it down, burying it near the house in a special spot where it could be seen, and marking the burial site with a rock or a piece of tin. Since the afterbirth had a special life force, any tampering

41

with it could compromise the mother's health. Using the afterbirth to manipulate spirits for positive or negative purposes is part of a number of practices and beliefs, some of them called "signs," common to southern blacks. Traditional Malaysian birth practices, like Nigerian ones, include puerperal roasting. Those who consider such customs as preparing the afterbirth with salt for protection and using sharp metal objects to ward off evil spirits as merely black superstition are ignoring the universality of these phenomena.

Some Alabama women rigorously enforced postpartum restrictions prohibiting extensive domestic and farm work. During this period, husbands often cooked for their wives and children, and grandmothers assisted with child care. Women and babies gained attention during ritualized "taking-up" ceremonies.

Ceremonies for the infant and for the reintegration of the mother into the daily routine varied, but the core of what Mrs. Smith practiced can also be found in the South Carolina Sea Islands and even, until recently, in some northern cities. The midwife might return for the taking-up ceremony, sometimes dressing the baby in a T-shirt made from flour sacks. She would carry the baby around the house three, seven, or nine times and name the baby. In bringing the baby into the light of the world, the midwife might sing, pray, simply talk to the Lord, and drink a thimble of water on returning to the house.

Mothers continued to rely on midwives and elder women in the community for support as their babies grew older. For teething problems a mother could string tread sash like beads around the baby's neck. Mothers might also place moles' feet in small bags around the child's neck upside down. Children could chew on the little bags when cutting teeth.

Respect for the elders' ways was a feature of black com-

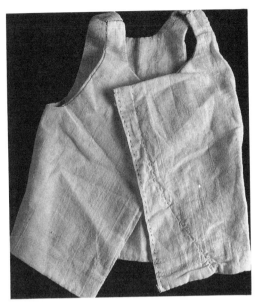

Infant's shirt made from flour sacks. Shirt courtesy of Bey Moten. Photo by Biggs Photography.

munities. The traditional system passed on by the elder women of the community included African elements, Native American practices, and standard medicine. Greene County's isolation and the fact that some of its inhabitants continued to pass on the birthing beliefs and customs orally, as they had received them, helped to sustain the old ways. During her own childbearing years, Mrs. Smith questioned the use of some of the teas prescribed by older midwives, and the rigidity of some birthing rules, but she complied with her grandmother's instructions. The prescriptions of her grandmother or other "old heads" in the community required no justification, for these women were seen as "wise women."

In the postpartum period, rest, some restrictions, dietary recommendations, and rituals made up the traditional way.

Initially, personal birth experience introduced younger women to the old-time birthing style. Later, teachings from the community's senior midwives through apprenticeships added greater specificity and depth to first-hand experience. Perhaps because women faced so much economic and political turmoil, passing on traditional ways became an important part of rising above subservience and establishing some cultural order. As Mrs. Smith says, "Those ways are just in me."

———————

I WAS A MESS WITH MY FIRST BABY. I said that man wasn't worth a shit nohow. That was the first man. I was about sixteen when the man got me pregnant. Oh, I hated that yellow bitch. Lord, I hated that man. He was the reason I got pregnant.

He said, "Margaret, let me and you marry."

I told that man, "I wouldn't marry you for nothing." I hated him worse than I hated a rattlesnake. I just didn't know I was getting a baby. I said, "No, you just go 'bout your business and I'll go 'bout mine." I met him at the church down there. I thought I was something, and let him sway me to do this.

He left here and married some woman up there. I didn't care what became of him. I didn't care if I never saw him no more. The only thing he ever gave the boy was fifty cents to buy him some candy.

I said, "I'm going to kill myself." I jumped off logs. I climbed trees. Thought I'd lose it. But the more I climbed, the bigger it got. I didn't want to sleep with Mama 'cause she might could tell about that baby in my belly. I told her I wanted a bed to myself, and she fixed a cot. My girlfriend stole me a sack, wrapped it like a girdle, and pinned it up on me in the woods, so you couldn't tell there was a baby in my belly. It was just that flat. I was scared, but I kept it. I stepped over in hell when I got a baby. But I said, I ain't staying with no man. I'm staying with my mama.

One Sunday, the old midwife had come to dinner. I was drawing water, toting water, and the midwife asked me did I have a baby in my belly.

I told her, "No ma'am."

But one night I woke up and Mama had pulled all the covers off me and found the sack.

She said, "What you doing with that sack? Are you big, Margaret?"

I said, "No ma'am."

She said, "I ain't going to beat you, but I tell you one thing, you got it, you going to have to work for it."

We were up in the mountains with the white people in Tennessee. It was summer. We used to go to Mount Eagle, Tennessee, in April till September, worked up there in the mountains. They have boarders come from different states, and there be one huge dining room and lots of bedrooms. We went early to clean up the cottages, put up the curtains. We helped cook, wait on tables, up there in the mountains. We took the train, changed in Chattanooga. They had a white coach and a colored coach.

At that particular time, I had to come back home because Mama was scared I might have that baby up there. Mama was the cook, and I was, you know, helping—make up beds, and wash bathrooms, clean and scrub, things like that. I think I came home this weekend and had the baby the next.

When I had that baby, I reared and bucked and carried on so they had to hold me down. I had a midwife, and it took me a few days to have it. That midwife came with a flour sack with

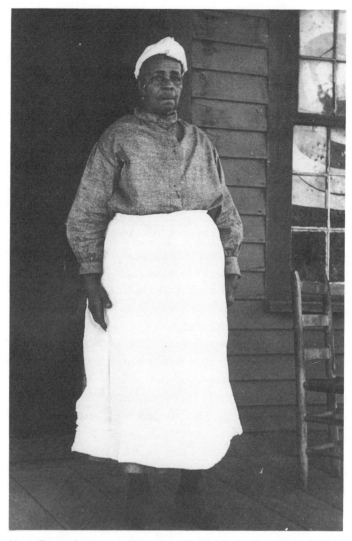

Aunt Dora Green, traditional midwife, Eufaula, Alabama, late 1930s. WPA Writers' Project, Alabama Department of Archives and History, Montgomery.

herbs in it to make teas. It was filled up to the top. She told me to put her on some water and boil it and make some tea.

I told her, "I wasn't able to drink the tea. There is no use in me drinking it and throwing it back up." Dirt dauber, black pepper seeped in a white cloth.

Then they put you in a tub of hot water, give you a hot bath and steam you up. If you weren't sick, you would be. They said it picked up the pains. If the pains cut off, they go and take kettles of boiling water, and they get it down to where you could sit in it, and steam you up again. They would have these babies before you knew it. Back in time, they didn't go by what the doctor said too much, 'cause there weren't any doctors.

I bucked with the first one pretty good. I just didn't know how to bear, and I just couldn't get myself in position to bear. Instead of bearing I raised and twisted a whole lot. I was down on the hard floor, and that floor was just killing me. I wasn't able to walk in about two weeks after that baby.

I wasn't married, and Mama didn't get there till two weeks after that. But she came, and I told her, "You can have it."

She said, "No, I'm going to keep you and the baby. But don't you go getting ne'er another."

I told her, "Don't worry. I won't."

People let children go haywire now, but back in them days, no sir. You didn't go anywhere. You weren't counted. You weren't recognized amongst the other girls when you became a mother.

After the baby came, I went back to work housecleaning. Mama said I got out there and got it, might as well get out there and work for it. And believe me, I did, too. I had two days a week. I had Saturday and Tuesday. Those were my days.

When we were having babies, there wasn't birth control. If there was, colored people didn't know anything about it. But some people just took things to keep from getting pregnant.

47

They have taken gunpowder out of a gun. I just didn't approve of that.

But I do remember them giving them teas to make their period come, and when they have cramps. They got some sort of root and gave it to them, but I never had complications with it. I heard Mama talk about it, talking to older women, her friends.

The second baby, I had that one by myself. I just got down. I liked that second man pretty good till he got that baby. Got here so my belly got to growing. My hips got to shaking like jelly.

I was staying in town, working in town. I just got down by the cot and put a quilt down. I went to my little room after I got through work. I did manage to work out. That day was Christmas Eve day and didn't have nothing but six apples and six oranges, had to get some sugar to make sweet bread just to know it was Christmas.

I said, "Lord have mercy, if I could just finish these white folks' dishes."

I just made it across the street to the room where I was staying. I crept on down that back street. That was one more creep. I hurt all day, and it turned over into evening.

When I made it there, I said, "Thank God, I done made it to the house." I threw down them things and put that quilt down with a pillow where I could put my arms up on it. And right there is where it happened. It wasn't over a half an hour before he was born. I don't know how I made it to my room. So there I was, me and the baby.

Sometimes it's a little longer till the afterbirth turns loose, but I was one that time wasn't long 'fore my afterbirth come. So I messed around until I had the afterbirth before I got up. Then I got me a piece of quilt and put it between my legs, and I took the baby and put him out from the placenta and propped his head up, and then I got back in the bed. I did it all myself.

My friend came, and she was hollering so. I told her what was happening, and she just started screaming. My friend went to the warehouse and called Dr. Moore. She had three children herself, but she was scared to death. She went and told my mama.

Dr. Moore was the midwife. We had no colored doctors. Some white doctors had colored nurses, but Dr. Moore was the old doctor. He cut the cord. I did the rest myself.

I'll tell you one thing, I'd rather be by myself. I didn't have any trouble that time, but see, I had been through it before. I just didn't want nobody putting me on the floor where I couldn't move. Some of them like the floor—not me. I wasn't a bit more scared, having the baby by myself.

When the doctor come, he told me I did a good job. I said to myself, "I know I've done a good one."

See, I was working for Kate, the postmaster of Eutaw. Kate was gone off somewhere. But when she got back and walked in the room and saw me, scared her to death.

She said, "Man, what the world you doing in the bed?"

I said, "Shit, I got a baby."

She said, "Who was here when it happened?"

"Nobody but me and the good Lord."


### The Elders' Ways

I stayed off six to seven weeks, and I came back home with my baby. They smoked your clothes when you got ready to get up, smoked them in the fireplace. When you got ready to go out on that third day, you smoked some cornmeal over it, if you got it.

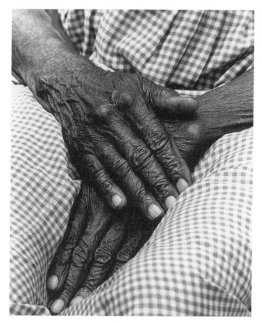

Hands of elderly midwife, Autauga County, 1981. Photo by Sharon Blackmon.

Put the cornmeal over the smoke. Let it smoke the clothes. Let it come up, let it smell like that smoke burned it. You have meal in the fire, about a handful and let it burn, then pass it over the fireplace or a wood stove. This would be the third day. Supposed to smoke your personal things, drawers, and the dress. If it's winter time, smoke the sweater.

My grandmother, the woman who raised me, smoked mine. When I had the one in town, she asked me if anybody smoked my clothes. I said no.

She said, "Well, I'm going to smoke them."

I took it. She said that it gives you strength where you weak at.

See, you have to be particular with the pieces with the blood on it. Now my mama washed mine. She wouldn't allow me to burn them. I brought them from Eutaw right over there. She washed them herself.

My baby was, I believe, it was two weeks old when they made me go around the house with the thimble of water. Mama brought me the thimble of water, and I had to carry it all the way around the house. Mama made me drink it when I got back. It was just a swallow. It wasn't a swallow. It was a little small thimble.

Then Mama said, "Well, now, when it's pretty and warm and dry and there's no rain when the dew dries off, you can go anywhere out here in this yard you want to, but you can't go out in the road or in somebody else's house."

I said, "Yes'm."

She told me I was supposed to do this. She never explained to me why, but you know she being an old person, I love to obey old people. So I just took the thimble of water and went on around the house.

When I got back, when I was coming back up the stairs she said, "When you get in the house, swallow that little swallow of water and put my thimble back."

So that's what I did. My baby was a month old before I went to cooking, and it was six weeks before I hit the ground. You couldn't go to field for six weeks to pick cotton 'cause the cotton was too white, it ruined your eyes. Everybody had cotton then, it looked like it done snowed in the field. My cousin came and cooked for me, but I was scared to eat fish, and no mustards, and no collards for six weeks, but you could eat turnips.

Mama always told me you could mark the baby in the first three months of pregnancy 'cause you might see a cow, dog, or

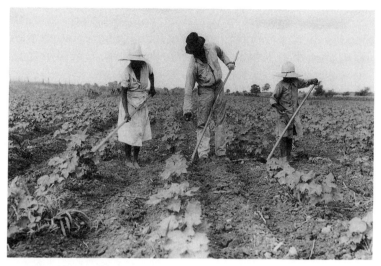

Family hoeing cotton, Eutaw vicinity, 1936. Photo by Dorothea Lange. Library of Congress Prints, U.S. Farm Security Administration.

something sick, hurt, hollering. On that account, you're not supposed to be around to pity it. But after the three months were up, you could go. That's what she said. After the first three months, then you're not as sensitive to those things.

When you are pregnant, you can eat just about anything you want. But after you had the baby, they told you to eat eggs, grits, things like that, but no fish. They wouldn't allow you to eat fish.

The one thing I took when I was pregnant was castor oil. I had to take castor oil. I took it, and I kept my stomach greased with it, but it's as nasty as it want to be.

The elder people back behind me had remedies that would help. People used to come to Mama for a lot of things. My grandmother used to give jimsonweed for fever. She'd get those weeds and pound them up, and they would be juicy like. Mama made a poultice and put it on your head where the hot area be.

When you are ready to have your baby, they used to give something like bamboo briar, that brings your pain on. You get that briar root in the field. You get the bottom part of the root when you pull the briar up. It has a root on it that's white, and you snip it. They cut it up in the joints. It's got a joint on it and they cut it up [upward motion] like that, and wash it right good and put on some water and let it be boiling and pour it over and get a saucer over that thing and you drink that stuff. Oh, it set your soul on fire!

Mayapple root was good because if it wasn't your time for you to have a baby, it would stop those pains. If it was time for that baby, they would bring the pains on. It comes from a crabapple bush, something like an apple tree, but it comes from the mayapple root. Little bitsy apples like they make jelly out of, women would get a root from it, just like it springs out from the tree, and wash it real good. You seep the briar root and boil the mayapple root. Make that tea and drink it like it is. And, then they used to make pepper teas. That would bring the pains on.

Tread sash is good for cleaning you out. It's real good with a cold. You have to cut it in those joints, wash it real good, put it on, let it boil, make a tea. Then take it off and put it in a cup and drink some when it gets past too hot.

Mama knew just about all the things to do for the baby. She grew catnip. She grew horehound, different stuff she grew in the garden, in the corner of the garden. People used to come 'cause she would be busy raising it. Everybody used to give the babies catnip, but for teething, Mama would say, get a man's band of his hat, cap, and cut you a little piece, big enough to go around that baby's neck. Another good thing is to get some cotton seed and bury them under the doorstep. Old folks had so many signs back then.

### Mama Died at 101

I just couldn't leave her. I never had the desire to leave her. That's the reason I was late in life marrying, because I just couldn't picture myself wanting to live somewhere and wanting to leave her. So I didn't. I just stayed right there . . . I just never could leave her. The more older I got the more I, you know, thought of her, the more I loved her, and I just couldn't leave her. I just didn't want to. The heck with marrying. I'll just stay with my mother. I just couldn't leave her. All the rest of them left but me. So I took care of her until she passed. I just couldn't leave her, wasn't going to leave her . . . I wasn't going to leave her. I thought too much of her. She's the only mother I know of. So why should I leave her? Nobody else to take her? But she wasn't sick long, from June to September . . . Never had but one child and raised ten of us, somebody else's children. She made us make a living, bet you that . . . I had to get out on my own. But I never did leave. I didn't mind as long as I could stay with her. You know, I always had the idea—I used to tell her when I was small if, when she died, I was going to die, too. They could put me in there with her. Hard times back in them days. I said after Mama passed, if I had paid attention to Mama, I wouldn't be slaving for nothing, raising children.

### Taking a Vow

I married Randolph Smith. I married him. We used to play together. We went to school together. I was late in life marrying. I was pretty close to my forties. I married him after Mama died.

We were chopping, chopping the second time, going over some cotton, when the last baby come. The midwife was working in the cotton field right over the fence in front of me. I chopped till I felt like I better quit. I quit and came on to the house.

The wagon brought the midwife over here, I think. That's where they found her, chopping cotton. The midwife had to go home and get her bag. Somebody took her home, but the baby was almost ready to be born. I didn't have but two pains and out the baby come. I had some newspaper down 'side the cot on the floor, and a woman called Nervie Carpenter was with me. I sent for her to come, and she come until we got hold of the midwife. I didn't have no choice that morning—I had to send for her.

She rubbed me. She'd just take my stomach, bring it to the front, and pull it down, and it look like those pains would kill me. I believe it was Vaseline, she rubbed my stomach with Vaseline, and she rubbed my back. She was all the help I had.

I had all the confidence in her. She was an older lady. I always did admire her. Anybody right around here, if she could walk, they would send for her, and she would go, if they were going to have a baby.

I told the midwife, "When I have the next one, you bet I won't have to call for you." I just needed a midwife to fill out the birth report. But after that, there weren't any more. I wanted a girl so bad, but I never did have an opportunity to get that girl. I thought waiting seventeen years for that last one, it might be a girl, then when I come up, fixing to get ready to go through my change, thinking I would have a girl, and it come out a boy, I could have cried. I just wanted a girl, but I had three boys.

## Reproductive Cycles

It was rough when I went through the change of life. I had clots. It looked like it was a baby's head falling into that slop jar bucket, a handful. But the best story is the running water, creek, or ditch. My mama's sister had thirteen children up here and she told me, "If you keep a-living, day will come, you gonna change."

I said, "Yes'm."

She said, "My best policy is to tell you while you changing not to have intercourse with a man too much because if you gonna knit back together, he gonna tear it a-loose and you going to continue. But the less you do that, the better off you are."

You know something up in there I imagine was closing back up, and she said "I'll tell you what you do. Whenever you start and know you in change of life, well and good, and the older person telling you, you changing, you straddle a ditch and get you a rag, and just like water running down and you straddling a ditch throw that water over you."

That's what I did. We got a big ditch going out from down here and I went down there two or three times just a-washing away. I said, "Lord have mercy."

It will go away and stay away for two or three months, but Lord when it do break loose again, you have to have a quilt. I ain't joking. You have to have a nice piece of quilt to soak up that blood. If not, it gonna come down your leg all over your bed, everywhere. Then it may go away and stay three or four months. Then it will come back. Keep on till you get through. Didn't nothing scare me but them clots. I went around the house. Folks didn't have toilets back then. And here come a big old drop of blood. Oh, Lord. I went to Miss Lucy Cockrell, and I asked her, and she said, "Oh shucks, Margaret, you ain't doing nothing but change of life."

I said "Ma'am."

She said, "Now you got to take care of yourself. You might not want to do it, but you just have to ease up off a man."

I said, "Yes'm."

And I said to myself, "Shit, I can go without seeing a man forever."

Children back in them days were ashamed to bring up a question at first, but I had to ask somebody what was the matter with me. Was I fixing to die, or did she know anybody that was in my shape?

She said, "Margaret, ain't nothing but your change in life."

I said, "Yes'm." I wanted to say, "Are you sure?" but I didn't say it. I just said, "Yes'm."

She said, "The only thing I can tell you is to lighten up off your boyfriend."

I said, "I can lighten up off him. Shit on a man. You get to the place where you rather be by yourself. Go to bed by yourself. Roll from one side of the bed to the other."

I tell you, it's a trip. It's a trip. I had a late change 'cause I got one boy right in front of the change. It's a trip. I can tell you that. That takes all the taste [for sex away] when you get through changing them pieces and try to go somewhere to let the clots go by, and there you sit. It's a trip. That's the last go, but you can get a baby during this thing right here.

## Farming

Long after Mama passed, I was still farming for me and the children. Sure did. A man ain't going to do nothing but mess you up nohow. You got to work for a man, or he wants to take all your money. You know men do that. I couldn't stand that. I had too hard of a time coming up for somebody to take my money. I sweated, and then I went to washing and ironing on top of that.

We had heard we was going to be broke up. That's what they mean when they take your stuff. I had seven head of cows, corn, plows, plow tools, and the man left me a basket of corn. I wasn't able to pay my bill for that year, and First National had went broke. See, that bank had to go out and get the stuff the mortgage called for. That broke me up, and do you know they took all the cows? They took seven head of cows, took the plow. What else did they take?

Oh, I said, "You can't get my hogs. No, you can't get them. Those don't go with the farm."

But they took my cotton seed and whatever. They took everything for the debt that you owed from before, and they left me a basket of corn.

They told me, "Don't you tell nobody. I'm leaving you a basket of corn."

We worked out to pay back the mules' time and the plowman. You either had to pick it out or chop it out. But the thing about it is when you go down there to the white man, he would ask you, "How much fertilizer you want?"

You tell him, "A ton or a ton and a half and two bushels or three bushels of cotton seed."

All right, that puts you on a piece of paper for the fall when you make that cotton. You can't sell it. You got to carry it to him.

This didn't just go for me. It went for a heap of people. The white people keep a colored person down because everything that he makes, they take it.

If you need a month's supply of groceries, you go down there and write your order, and you carry it over there to such-and-such a man's store. He filled the order. Nothing but slavery.

I worked for the mule and plow. I chopped a day, me and that oldest boy of mine, for the mule and plow—a day. That's the way I got on up, working. Plowed like a man with mules. The children hated going to field, but they had to go.

If the white man was giving an advance, they would really come out to make sure you were out in the cotton field. One good year, we raised a good bit of cotton. I raised five bales that year. We would pick cotton at night in the moonshine. Moon would be shining pretty in the rows. Wasn't no grass in the field. You could just go out there and help yourself, picking, picking by the moonlight, a many a hundred pounds of cotton we picked at night.

We planted cotton in April and it goes to opening in August. Buddy, that sun looked like it would eat you up. You could see monkeys dancing in the field.

One March after we settled, the white man told Randolph, if he had just made one more bale of cotton, he would have come out even. Well, that's when I cussed and raised hell. I cussed Randolph out, that is what I done. When it was time to go back to field, I told him I wasn't going. I was going to hunt me a job, which I did.

I said, "My children can make it, and I'm going to make it. They're barefoot, and I'm barefoot. We didn't have clothes to put on our backs. No sir, I ain't going back, not now."

I told Randolph that I've done all I'm going to do, and I meant that. "I ain't going to work not another lick in nobody's field."

I just told him, "I'm going to look for a job. If I get a start again, no Mr. White Man is going to come up here to tell me he wants my things."

I had my house, and my husband had his house way over yonder. Some days I'd cook over there to his house. He had his own house 'cause he had been married once before. We lived in the same house when night come. He come over here 'cause I had to be where my children were. I couldn't leave them over here beside the road and I'm back over there behind on that side. He lived over across the creek. It wasn't his house. He rented that place. I'd cook breakfast at home for my children, and we'd all eat, and I'd carry his breakfast over there to him.

I was working in the field now. I wasn't missing that. He wasn't getting nothing. He was just working on his debt that he owed. Wasn't no money to come unless you planted out your cotton, you might come out ahead. Let's say I had two bales of cotton. They sold it for so much a pound. Some cotton sold for ten cents a pound. Some sold for fifteen cents, and like that. It didn't get higher to time commenced to getting a little better. He was plowing over there and plowing over here on my farm, too. See, he took the biggest portion of plowing off me. See, I helped him some days. And some days I wouldn't, but I just quit helping him for awhile. I didn't see where I was doing him no good, and I had to make it some way or another.

### Domestic Work

Then I messed around and went back to work for the postmaster of Eutaw and thought she was paying me good. Sometimes she gave the children clothes, and that helped. I'd walk from right over there to Eutaw to work and come back. I sweated, and then I went to field on top of that. In the evening, while I was still at the job, I had to wash them chairs on the front porch. I had to scrub the porch off and put those chairs back when they dried. They had pretty flowers, and I had to get down on my knees after dinner and pull that wild grass. They had a cement walk on each side, I had to pull wild grass out the flowers on each side of the walkway. They also had big leaves from those magnolia trees to be swept up.

You ironed sheets then. Iron them on both sides. Fold them correct, too. Iron those pillowcases, starched. And they say, "My summer dresses, starched!"

Lord! Set up so many Friday nights till one and two o'clock ironing. Get up next morning milk, cook, hit the road going to Eutaw to work with a basket of clothes on my head, icicles popping up on the side of the road. Sometimes people would pick me up, and sometimes they didn't, but I kept on till I got some changing clothes. This day, I get one son a little suit. Now I'm still leaving myself off 'cause they had to go to school, and I didn't want them to go looking like tramps.

Sometimes I felt so sorry for my husband. He's out there, be plowing. When he got tired of plowing, he'd go to chopping. I'd get the hoe on the weekends, on Saturday, and I'd help him out. My husband and I like to quit when I first started working 'cause I had to come to the house and fix him some dinner, if I didn't fix it overnight. Sometimes I would, and sometimes I'd be so tired I couldn't.

I got to the place I was going everywhere. I was staying away from home too long with a family. You have to be with a family. You can't be away from it. In a portion, my husband didn't mind. In a portion, he just didn't want me to do. But I did it anyway because I had to have some cash money. My children had to have clothes, shoes, decent food. He was working in the field. That was the only place people had to work at till the CWA came along. And then they started giving fifty cents an hour sanding the roads, putting sand on the road. The boys were getting on up, big boys. They didn't like the field. They knew if they picked that cotton that they could help me get some money so they could get shoes, at least some clothes, you know, to change in. I don't know how many times I made me a fire at night and washed their underwear and hung it to the fire. One of the boys, he quit school 'cause he didn't have no really nice breeches like he really wanted to wear every day. You know the city boys. He was wearing the yellow khaki breeches and that made him sick and he quit.

That same year, when it was time to go to field, the white man come back and asked me, "Where's Randolph?"

I said, "I don't know where he's at. In the field, I reckon."

He said " How come you ain't out there chopping?"

That's when I told that white man off.

I said, "I've been helping Randolph work on his bill for four or five years, and I ain't got nothing. I was naked, my children were naked. I done got me a job."

The white man told Randolph I was crazy. I said, "No, I ain't crazy. I just told the white man what I wasn't going to do. I know he can't make me do 'cause I didn't have a debt. I was helping you 'cause you are my husband."

I said, "I don't give a hoot what comes of the field. I figured we made five bales of cotton. The white man got that. I figured we had to come out of debt, and we'd have a little money. Shoes then was cheap, two dollars, a dollar fifty a pair. You could get some shoes.

# | 3 |

# OFFICIAL MIDWIFE

*In officiating at births,* women employed talents that the constant drudgery of farm and day work never allowed to come out. Working as midwives, they took on significant responsibilities. Many of the midwives I interviewed saw themselves as "poor people who missed an opportunity to pursue an education," but they went on to say that midwifery put their "big minds" to work. While taking pride in their abilities to plow like men, split rails like men, and pick cotton by the moonlight, these women found in midwifery a diversion from weary subservience, a break from mindless menial labor, and a chance to use their skills in ways that benefited women in their communities.

In the early twentieth century, the Children's Bureau of the U.S. Department of Labor began to investigate the problem of maternal and infant mortality. The studies they sponsored linked the deaths of mothers and babies to problems of poverty, lack of prenatal care, lack of access to health care facilities, and poor medical practices. While failing to address the economic, political, and social problems that lay at the heart of the matter, Alabama officials made some efforts to increase access to prenatal care and to regulate midwives.

Doctors were never scrutinized like midwives, despite findings that white women receiving private medical care had higher maternal and infant mortality rates than poor and rural black women going to prenatal clinics and having midwife-supported births. For example, Jessie L. Marriner, director of public health nursing, in 1928 recognized that midwifery was a "time-honored institution in Alabama," but she joined with other authorities in depicting midwives as the cause for many maternal and infant care problems and worked hard to institute a system for formal training and registration of midwives. Since the majority of midwives only occasionally attended births, Marriner recommended focusing midwife control programs on the less than 25 percent of the midwives who attended 70 percent of midwife births. The inability of such programs to validate self-taught women and their important cultural practices ultimately drove some of the most active women out of midwifery and led others to experience a loss of autonomy. Even as the women learned more, training programs emphasized limiting their practices.

A 1918 state law requiring that midwives pass an elementary examination and register under the State Board of Health had prompted the Andrew Memorial Hospital to offer its services as a training site for Alabama's black midwives. Of the fifty midwives who entered the program that year, forty-three completed the course, which emphasized simple hygiene and such domestic skills as making beds, preparing foods, and giving baths. Thousands of women practiced as midwives in Alabama, but only a handful completed the Tuskegee program in its early years. For the next several decades, health care professionals would distinguish midwives with exposure to official training from those who learned mostly from experience and community apprenticeships. No matter how short or disparate the formal training program, trained midwives gained favor with professional health care providers. Many of the trained Tuskegee midwives also enjoyed increased status in their communities, although some women preferred the untrained birth attendant. In the early years of the program, Dr. Kenney of Andrew Memorial Hospital observed: "It was interesting to see these women, some in their seventies, many of whom had never attended school a day in their lives, coming back and forth daily for their instruction. They were very enthusiastic over the work given them" (8).

In 1931 there were 3,568 midwives in Alabama under the supervision of county health departments in fifty-four of the sixty-seven counties. Midwives "waited on" most of the births in the black community, and, most dismaying to medical authorities, midwives increasingly attended births in the white community as well, perhaps a reflection of both the deepening economic problems of the depression years and the preference for midwives. Writing in a 1935 issue of the *Alabama Medical Transactions*, A. E. Thomas complained, "The midwife problem becomes more pernicious as the years roll by. We reported last year that the number of mothers taken care of by midwives was on the increase, and we regret to say it continues to increase" (148). In other issues of the *Alabama Medical Transactions*, doctors ridiculed midwives for their dialect and their methods, such as the use of a cloth drenched in spiderwebs to induce clotting, but seldom assessed the efficacy of any of these techniques.

Over the course of the twentieth century, Alabama women gained increased access to maternity care, health care professionals, and some trained midwives. By 1944 findings of the Alabama Bureau of Maternal and Child Health indicated that 12 percent of Alabama women attended clinics. White women accounted for only 2.3 percent of that population, as clinic care was viewed a last resort for poor blacks and a federal imposition of socialized medicine. Yet the bureau's quality-of-care study showed positive outcomes for women enrolled in prenatal clinics. The *Alabama Medical Journal* concluded: "If we take the two opposite

**THE ALABAMA LEGISLATURE PROVIDED**

that every citizen between the ages of 14-50 shall have a blood test for

# SYPHILIS

The State Department of Health has designated Feb. 24 thru March 7, except Saturday and Sunday as the time for making this test in Greene County.

Blood Testing Stations have been arranged in practically every community in the county, as designated below. Please study these Stations and arrange to be present at one of them.

1. The law provides a fine for those failing to report.

2. Trained and certified nurses and doctors will serve the county.

3. A team of investigators will follow this test and check records and census files for delinquents. The law will be enforced.

4. In case of illness one may have his test delayed by getting a certificate from his physician to this effect. The law then places the responsibility for this test on the physician

### THE COOPERATION OF EVERY PERSON IS REQUESTED.

Signed:

H. MONTGOMERY, Probate Judge
K. SMITH, Mayor Eutaw
FRANK LEE, Sheriff

S. D. BAYER, County Superintendent of Education
DR. S. J. WILLIAMS, County Health Officer
DR. D. G. GILL, State Health Officer

BLOOD TESTING SCHEDULE FOR GREENE COUNTY

MONDAY FEBRUARY 24th THROUGH FRIDAY MARCH 7 1947

**EUTAW (WHITE)**
COURT HOUSE ROOM—Wednesday, February 26th through Thursday, February 27th—8:30 AM to 4:30 PM

**EUTAW (COLORED)**
COURT HOUSE COURT ROOM—Monday, February 24th through Tuesday February 25th—8:30 AM to 4:30 PM

Announcement for blood testing, February 20, 1947, *Greene County Democrat.*

extremes economically and educationally, namely, the white (non-clinic) patient and the colored clinic patient, it is rather startling to find the colored rate is lower than the white in maternal mortality by 9 percent and neonatal mortality by 35 percent, but higher in stillbirths by 13 percent, probably in the main because of the prevalence of syphilis in the colored."

Prenatal care may have improved, but racial inequities and abuses continued. A blood-testing program for syphilis at nearby Tuskegee led to human rights violations, including denial of medical treatment to those suffering from the disease. The high incidence of syphilis in Alabama's black population heightened stereotyping about black sexual behaviors. Anti-midwife efforts continued to be clouded by attitudes of racial superiority. In the 1940s, white doctors specifically targeted white women in campaigns to drive them away from black midwifery care. Title V of the Social Security Act brought new funds for child health clinics and midwife training programs to the state. The Alabama State Health Department also used some of its federal dollars to add personnel to state and county health departments. Greene County opened a health office in 1937; its first project was the examination of all schoolchildren.

In the late 1940s Mrs. Smith became one of Greene County's official midwives. After years of helping out at births for relatives, she obtained a permit when recruited by local physicians, trained, and registered. Unlike the other dozen or so practicing midwives with permits who never became a part of the public health team in Greene County, Mrs. Smith worked regularly in public health prenatal clinics.

The Alabama Board of Health criteria for selection included good Christian morals and indications of personal and domestic cleanliness. Alabama required that midwives have two recommendations from local doctors, who then had to document their support of individual midwives through annual renewals of midwife permits. Need may also have played a part in Mrs. Smith's selection, because in 1946 the local public health registrar, Mrs. Jeanie Bayer, had noted a need to "replace the one who died a few months ago." That year, the Eutaw registrar listed the names of three physicians, Joe P. Smith, Don Smith, and R. S. Lucious, and two midwives, Mollie Colvin and Ida Colvin.

For new midwife recruits, the Greene County Health

Department offered a month-long Saturday training course. The women also attended the special statewide Tuskegee lay-midwife program. At Tuskegee, lay midwives gained clinical experience in the maternity unit of Andrew Memorial Hospital, where rural women with medical complications received care at a cost of ten dollars for a ten-day stay.

In addition to its well known lay-midwife program, Tuskegee developed a nurse-midwife program, which lasted only a few years because of difficulty in recruiting faculty and attracting students, who preferred schools in more cosmopolitan locations with fewer racial tensions. There was some respect between nurse-midwives and their lay counterparts, but even some of the most supportive public health nurses and nurse-midwives refused to recognize the empirical skills of lay midwives.

Midwives like Mrs. Smith took their new training into their souls, but they also used skills and knowledge they had acquired in apprenticeships with community midwives. While sometimes counting on miracles in a crisis, Mrs. Smith recognized that her skills were the bottom line. Training emphasized reliance on medical backup, but midwives had to be self-reliant because they faced old barriers: institutional segregation, gender discrimination, and professional elitism. Their cooperation with physicians and nurses in the public health system was not rewarded with full respect or support. Alabama's lay midwives remained trapped at the bottom of the social and medical hierarchy.

---

MY HUSBAND'S FIRST COUSIN'S WIFE [Louise] used to live right straight up on that hill from here. I'm telling you, there's nothing there now but the old well. And she had thirteen

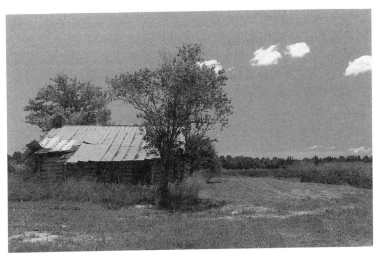

Abandoned cabin, Greene County, 1995. Photo by Sharon Blackmon.

children. I being right here, she would come out—wasn't any pine trees or nothing growing there—she would come out and call me, and I could hear her. She'd tell me to come there, and I'd go. Every time she would have a baby, I'd be there.

See, her husband didn't like her to visit with people. You know how some men are. They are jealous, and they just didn't want anybody hanging around. They were afraid they might get their wife. I was the only somebody within the family right down the hill from her that he didn't mind. She would come down and borrow things and get things, and I would go up there, 'cause he didn't allow no other women there but me. Her husband would bring my groceries from town on the mule. He worked in town. He'd do things for me and Mama, and that was a help.

See, I always thought I should benefit myself some, but the Lord wants you to do good things to help other people. That's what the Lord wants, help the needy, and she was in need. Nobody to be with her.

I'm so flip. Every time she would get in labor, they send for me. I'd be there till her husband go to, say, Clinton or go to Eutaw to hunt a midwife. Well, in the meantime, here comes the baby.

So I bumped into Miss Ella Anderson when she was coming down to the ninth child, I think it was. Miss Ella says, "Uh, Margaret, why don't you be a midwife?"

I say, "No Lord, uh-uh. I'm not going to be a midwife." But she just kept a-worrying me, every time.

Louise would have a baby every year. When Miss Ella Anderson come, I be done got the baby. You know, got me a string and tied the cord to keep the blood from running out the baby. I'd stop it till the midwife got there.

My brother-in-law, he had twelve, and I delivered six of his children. My other brother-in-law had over thirteen in Springfield. I delivered half of them. They are all living right now, right over there, what's here.

So it rocked on down until Louise had some difficulty in the thirteenth child. She commenced to bleeding so much before the baby come.

I said, "Lucius, you better get up from there, son, and go get the doctor, the midwife, or somebody. Your wife is bleeding too much."

He said, "Well, probably just that gonna be."

I said, "No, I don't think it is."

In the meantime, I run down the hill to my house and called the doctor.

He says, "Is it bad?"

I say, "Yes sir, it's pretty bad."

So the doctor and me and Miss Ella Anderson were up

there at the same time. All three of us there, one right behind another.

The doctor said if he hadn't got there, she would have lost too much blood in front of the baby.

I said to myself, "Yep, thought that."

That's something she never did, lost that much blood. As fast as I could put a towel or piece of quilt under her, the quilt would be wet before you know anything, just soaking wet. You could just wring the blood out. She was on up in age, too, when she had the last child.

That's when the doctor said, "Why don't you go and be a midwife?"

I said, "No sir. I don't want to be a midwife. I can't be none. No sir, nobody's going to turn me into a midwife."

He said, "Well, I am."

I said, "No sir, not me. Don't you turn me in."

But he did anyway. I just didn't want to be a midwife. I didn't want to be one because I saw what Miss Ella Anderson had to go through with, and how she had to travel. Transportation was somewhat scarce here. When you see a car, that was a big thing. Me and her would get out at night. You know it wasn't dangerous then. Wasn't no cars like it is now. We would walk to places. It was a horse, buggy, mule or buggy, or wagon, and I rode in a many of one of them at night, going through the waters, snow, and ice. The other part didn't worry me, just the transportation. I saw how she had to go and what she had to go through with, the good and the bad.

I said, "Uh-uh, no."

Stay away from home all night and no coffee the next morning. Nowhere to wash your face, and you look like you've come out the sewer pipe.

I said, "No, Miss Ella. Your transportation ain't right."

There were seventeen of us [midwives] when I started my midwife work. I was the last midwife in Greene County to get a permit. I went three months around here on Saturdays at their health department. They had the trained nurses at the health department, and we had a group of midwives this Saturday and another group the next Saturday, but not many people would come.

In those classes, the nurses sat on one side of the room and the midwives on the other. We were doing most of the colored births in Greene County. The midwives who would come took part in the training on Saturday morning from eight o'clock to eleven o'clock for three months. Those classes were during the summer months. Our teacher, Miss Jones, she thought midwives were great. White midwives were in the state that she was in.

They be asking you questions: "How can you tell when the baby crowns?"

You know, anybody can tell when the baby crowns. Baby's fixing to come here then—fixing to bust on out and get here.

After those classes, you come to meetings twice a year and bring your midwife bag in. They had to check your bags. You had a thing made inside your bag with some pockets in it for different items to go in—your scissors and a tray, your scales, your orange sticks, and your soap, your cap, and your mask. Your mask was made out of yellow domestic. Down at the bottom, they had a big place to put your gown. You carried eyedrops, the cord dressings, and scales. Then they had a drawstring to pull to make it look like a pocketbook.

The real big thing came off when they sent me to Tuskegee. I stayed over there two weeks until the day we came back. The head nurse carried a load of us for the special two-week training. Midwives out of Tuscaloosa, Demopolis, over three hundred of us there together, and those rooms were hot. We stayed in the nursing dorms up there. At that time they didn't have no fans, no nothing. They had all kinds of things we could work with, like dolls with the string coming out their stomach. We had to cut and tie that off, and see how well we did. We examined the afterbirth, the placenta, I would say. They just kept asking us questions. Every day we went to the hospital. Every time somebody over in the hospital would have a baby, they would take a bunch of us over, every day. We would put a mask on and just sit back and watch. If we didn't go to the hospital, they would send the afterbirth over there to us.

### Hard Times

Listen to me good. Back when I started, it was kind of poor. At that time, the people didn't have nothing. You couldn't get nothing. They had to do the very best they could. Some of them didn't have places to sit. They didn't even have a piece of white sheet, clean or nothing. I'd have to get up sometime and go to the next-door house and ask her to give me some clean rags, if she had 'em. Just barely living.

I wouldn't say the people couldn't work, 'cause listen, you could pick up pecans in the wintertime, and they pay you so much a pound or bushel or what in ever you picked up or either they give you pecans, and you could sell them or either you could go somewhere to pick cotton, if you could pick it. But if you couldn't pick cotton, it wouldn't be necessary for you to go. Some people just couldn't pick it, and some people could. Well, it be so hot. If you walked from here to out yonder and tried to pick a hundred pounds of cotton, you ain't much good. See, they put you on a piece of paper. Everybody knew their place. You would go down to Eutaw and they would ask

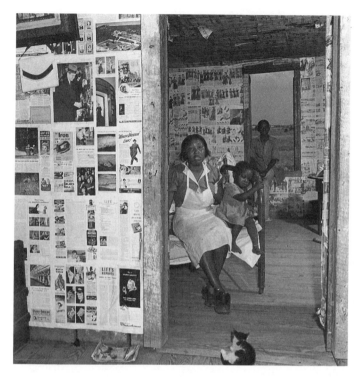

Tenant family at home in their newspaper-walled house, 1941. Photo by Jack Delano. Library of Congress Prints, U.S. Farm Security Administration.

you how much fertilizer you want. You would tell them and then say two or three bushels of cotton seed. All right, that put you on a piece of paper. For the fall when you make that cotton, you can't sell it. You got to take it to him. He does the selling.

There's still cotton now, but you can't get no job picking cotton. Machines pick it now. Cotton went before the midwife because they got these machines in, and people didn't have those jobs and didn't have to pick. And the next thing they got was a corn puller. Folks used to have to pull the corn. Cockle-burs up over your head. Water licking off the hem of your dress. That was hard time, I call it, back then. People lived in newspaper houses, I would say, with flour holding it together.

So this is the way I began. I started out with the lady who would come and take care of Louise, named Ella Anderson. I would go with her in spare chances, taking this job up and keeping on. I went on a year or better with Miss Ella Anderson. She lived four miles up on top of that hill.

I took training courses, but the midwife had already trained me, Ella Anderson. I learned everything, learned how to ask the mother if she was ready—does she have all her equipment ready? You know—the newspaper, something to boil the water in, something for the baby. But you just didn't need nothing new for the baby. Somebody else may have some things you could borrow or use. See what I mean? But every-thing, everything I learned, I learned from Miss Anderson. See, Miss Ella Anderson had done learned me, and I didn't forget it. Some of the other midwives thought they were the master of birds around here, but I learned from Miss Ella Anderson. She was just a kindhearted person. Miss Ella Anderson, I think she quit. I don't think she liked the new law. They were always tell-ing us what the mothers had to have and what they had to do. They were real strict on us, too.

I said to myself, "Well, shit, can't nobody prepare what they don't have."

Regardless of how it was, we had to go through it 'cause we took that oath saying that we would. Didn't care if it wasn't clean. Didn't care how it was, you had to go through it or you had to give an accounting or one. That's another thing that I disliked about it, the strict law they had on us and no pay. They didn't have no law to make them pay us. See, the nurses at the health department set the prices we got paid. It started off at five, then it went to ten, to fifteen, to twenty. When it got on up there to fifty, that's when they wanted the midwives off.

Some of the children, I meet them now, they've grown and gone. Mama ain't never paid me, Daddy ain't never paid me. I just give it to them. I'm short.

Back then, if I asked you, and you know you owe me and say, "Well, Margaret, you come to town tomorrow. Be there at twelve o'clock or eleven o'clock. I'm going to pay you."

Well, here I go just click, click, click, walking all over town. Never see a person. I reckon I be worn out that week delivering babies, and I see everybody in the world but you, 'cause you owe me.

They say, "Well, Miss Margaret, you be sure to be in Eutaw Saturday. I get my check, and I'll be there."

That was my money. If I came here last night and waited on you, and you paid me that ten or twenty when it was up there, twenty-five dollars, that was my gain. That money was mine. There were so many things I needed. That was my spending money.

Got me to the place that I don't want to go to Eutaw on Saturday now. I was walking round there like I was drunk on whiskey—peeping, looking, see if I could see that fellow that owed me. When I see him, he had a great excuse.

### Regular Paycheck

It wasn't no time when I started working part-time at the health department. I worked a year for nothing. All of the other midwives who started quit the health department except for me. They figured they weren't getting anything. After I took the oath to be a midwife, I just decided to stay on and do what they said.

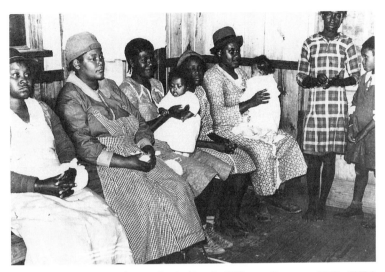

Women waiting in clinic, Gee's Bend, Wilcox County, 1939. WPA Alabama Writers' Project, Alabama Department of Archives and History, Montgomery.

I worked at the clinic twenty-eight years before I left. They had prenatal care, and the ladies would meet at these different clinics which were nearest to them. Then we'd go that morning for them to do the blood work, get the urine, and do different things on them. I had them up on the table, and the doctor would examine them.

They had this big clinic where they were taking care of, mostly what they were taking care of was colored people. They had a clinic here, one in Boligee and one in Tishibe. See, I worked at all three of the clinics. I worked in Boligee on Friday. Worked in Tishibe on Thursday. Worked in Eutaw on Tuesday. Every Tuesday that come round that week, that was my day to work. If I didn't get through that day, I'd have to

77

go back there Wednesday 'cause I had all the specimen to clean and all.

I sterilized the needles and everything. I had all that to do and get up the laundry. I did all the washing and cleaning and fixed up the tables for the next Tuesday. They had the cloth gown with just the strings to tie around you, but they had to be washed. I had the towels to wash. I had to sterilize them. We had the roll of paper to put under the bottom of the women, and we had the sheets to put over them. So I had them to wash. Then I had all those speculum that you put up in there to spread them open with. I had them to wash. Then I had a whole bunch of syringes and needles to wash.

I also helped to get the ladies into the clinic to keep their appointments. I tried to make sure they got in somehow or another. See, they don't allow midwives to deliver unless the doctor writes out a statement. My name is signed to the bottom of the card. You can't go unless they bring the paper to you first. Then you have the paper, and the doctor signed it. I'd been trained all along not to fool with somebody unless the doctor O.K.'d the paper stating that the patient is O.K. for a midwife.

I worked at the clinic with the pregnant ladies, and they knew me. They had to put on the gowns and things and get ready. I'd be standing right 'side the head of the examining table, and the doctor at the other end. After knowing me, they wanted to make a special trip to my house or either see me in town somewhere and tell me they wanted me to wait on them. That's how my name spread.

I'd tell them all the time that if the clinic gives them a paper stating it's O.K. to have a midwife, I'd be glad to deliver them, but if the doctor didn't O.K. them, I couldn't. They knew that up front.

## Born Dead

The first baby I delivered was a stillborn, like to scare me to death. This was after I'd done took the oath and got my permit, going out as a licensed midwife. I think it still affects my heart in this day now.

My folks lived over there in Pine Grove. Laura Kate married some of my folks, brother B.'s boy, and that caused us to be in the family. She married a Smith, and I did too. She married a brother, and I married a brother. It was two brothers. So I was scared of dead people, and Lord, I never will forget that stillborn. I never been out on delivery on my own by myself. That was my first delivery.

You know they trained us, the midwife, if the woman didn't go to the clinic, but to the doctor, we are supposed to go to the doctor with the card from the health department, and ask the doctor about the patient, and he's supposed to tell us what's happening.

So I went to the doctor, and he told me, "Yes, she's hurting, and she's going to have a baby, but I'll tell you one thing, the baby was living up to two weeks ago."

He hadn't seen her for two weeks, but he said, "The baby is going to be dead when he's born."

I said, "Yes, sir."

I know he saw my complexion change when he said, "He's going to be dead."

Then the doctor told me, "All you got to do is go there and wait till the baby comes. That's all you got to do, and bring the birth certificate by me."

I said, "Yes sir," but I like to die.

Then he told me, "You got to dress him."

That's when I said, "I'm sorry, but I can't do that."

79

He told me, "This is your job to go through with it."

I said to myself, "I know one thing. I'm going to give these people's delivering stuff back to them. I'd rather go to field than be a midwife. I can't fool with dead folks."

The doctor said, "And there ain't no use to keep on coming around here and worrying me. Just go ahead and catch it." Well, I like to have a heart attack. I think it still affects my heart in this day now.

When the baby come, I was sweating just big drops of sweat, trying to bathe this baby—put the baby on the quilt. You could look up in that house and see the stars. The wind was blowing, but that was all right 'cause I was still dropping big beads of sweat.

You know you always have your clean rag or something to help the baby out with. I thought that B. or Tip or some of them were going to take over and swathe the baby. So, fast ass Tip just hopped up and said, "Well, I know one thing . . ." Tip was the auntie of the boy who married Kate.

I looked up quick to catch on.

I said, "What you say?"

She said, "Well, you got this job, and you got to swathe this baby."

They said they did it 'cause it broke me up from being scared. I had to try to bathe that baby and had to try to put some clothes on him, a little dress, a little gown, or whatever, to bury him in. My lap across here was just trembling. I could feel the coldness from my baby on my thighs. And they were just killing themselves laughing. They could see I was scared to death.

I was so glad when day broke, I didn't know what to do. I was so scared, Lord, I was so scared. Well, I commenced to thinking, and Tip, she was older than any of them up there in the house, she just kept a-talking to you.

Tip said, "Margaret, you had no business taking it, and now that you done took it, and this is your first trip, you should serve a year anyway and make the best of it you can. The dead ain't going to hurt you."

I said, "Yeah, Tip, but I can't stand it."

She said, "Yes, you can. You can go through with it. That's why we wanted to help you, to break you in."

I said, "Tip, I tell you, I done made a great mistake in life."

She said, "No, you ain't. You doing what the Lord wants you to do. Now if you weren't doing what the Lord wanted you to do, you wouldn't have knowledge enough to do it. You didn't do this on your own—the Lord willed this, for you to do this kind of work and try to make the best of it you can, 'cause the dead ain't going to bother you."

But I prayed to God that I ne'er deliver a baby or a woman like that one. I had to dress several more babies, but I wasn't scared 'cause Tip made me take my hand and rub it over that baby's face.

# | 4 |

# BIRTH PRACTICES

*Midwives excel in* ushering in normal and healthy births, and many of Alabama midwives' practices are models in the field. These include keeping the mother active as long as possible during labor; helping the mother feel strong enough to endure labor through relaxation, comfort, and support; respecting a mother's ability to birth her own baby; supporting a woman's birth in a familiar setting; rubbing and massaging a woman as needed in pregnancy and in labor; encouraging alternative (upright) birthing positions; delaying cutting of the umbilical cord; keeping mother and baby together as much as possible right after birth; encouraging breast-feeding; and limiting the use of technological and pharmaceutical interventions.

### Normal Births

Not surprisingly, many midwives described their roles as witnessing births, not managing deliveries. Midwives told women: "Let nature take its course," "When the apple is ripe it will fall," and "A baby's got to come on its own time, honey." This way of thinking led midwives to encourage women in labor to "keep a-stumbling, keep a-moving, doing something, if it ain't nothing but walking, stirring around." Midwives also physically supported a mother as she entered the last stage of labor and pushed the baby out. As Dr. J. J.

Kirschenfeld, a rural doctor in Lowndes County, Alabama, recalled in his autobiography, *No Greater Privilege*, "Several times I was astonished to find a midwife in bed with the mother (black or white), feet to feet, for more effective bearing down."

Some rural physicians' practices had more in common with midwife practices than with hospital-based obstetrics. In the 1940s, country doctors increasingly depended on forceps and made use of anesthesia and pitocin in the home, but others favored a natural approach. They took pride in their abilities to manage without hospital nurseries or nurses and left sterile caps, masks, and gowns for hospital use. And, like midwives, some country doctors attended births for little pay in small cabins off country dirt roads with no lights or running water. Because of their status as physicians, however, they were able to make their case for residential deliveries in the pages of the state medical journal and to inform their peers that these deliveries could be as successful as those performed in the hospital.

Midwives had no such way to promote their practices and record their successes. Instead, community members had to speak for them, testifying to their skills and to their spirituality. Mothers recalled the willingness of midwives to remain with them throughout labor and birth in spite of lengthy labors and uncomfortable home settings. As Herlene Pipping, a neighbor of Mrs. Smith's, recalled: "At that time, the midwife would stay, if it took two or three days, that black midwife would be there. Midwives at that time had hard times. They had a good heart. So many midwives are dead and gone and didn't get nothing. Sitting up all night long, the door cracked, spread a quilt down, I'm telling you, it be rough. But God always has a way to bring his children out." Another Greene County resident, Augusta Duncan, summed it up this way: "Couldn't no doctor in town or

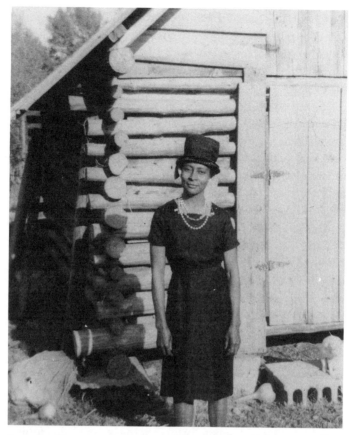

Augusta Duncan in front of Mrs. Smith's smokehouse after Randolph Smith's funeral, c. 1967. Photo courtesy of Augusta Duncan.

anywhere else could of made me feel any better than Mrs. Smith in assuring me that everything was going to be all right, and it was."

Midwives often demonstrated the spiritual dimension of their work during labor and birth. They described to me "putting God ahead," "taking the Lord into their insides," "having some kind of feeling knowing they are always blessed," "not working with nothing unless God is in it," and having "much communication with the spirit" as part of the philosophy that infused all their acts. Others said that they could "count on God to get to the birth before they did," "to be the doctor," and to show them signs before complications occurred.

### Social Realities

Widespread poverty meant that midwives often struggled to create birthing pallets from torn quilts and rags. They delivered women living in shacks without window coverings and running water. Poverty led to overwork, poor diets, closely spaced births, and harsh living conditions, causing major health problems among women giving birth.

Practices like geophagy (also found in West Africa) were common in the rural South and influenced birth outcomes. Descriptions of cravings for white and red clays can be found in the medical literature. Midwives told me about women who ate sour dirt, "tangy and cheese-like," sometimes enhanced by salting or heating. Midwives understood the practice, but sometimes expressed dismay over having to attend births where the babies appeared to be covered with the earthy substance because of a mother's indulgence.

Poor rural counties with large black populations typically had few physicians. In 1949, T. M. Boulware, chairman of the Alabama Medical Society's Maternal and Child Health Committee, reported that Greene County was one of five counties in Alabama with the greatest need for physician assistance. The state medical society urged the five counties to resolve the problem by paying white physicians to provide indigent care and by looking to regionalized black higher

education as a way to increase the number of black professionals, but this recommendation had little effect. Black residents of Greene and other counties depended on the services
offered at Tuskegee's Andrew Memorial Hospital, nearly
two hundred miles from Eutaw. While the black community
respected Tuskegee's services, many could not get to this
black medical institution. Local maternity clinics in Greene
County sometimes had nurses drive women to Tuskegee. At
other times the Gandy Funeral Home hearse (funeral homes
commonly provided emergency transportation) was the only
way to get to a hospital. Greene County families respected
Tuskegee's midwife training programs, saw the institution
as a beacon of self-help and a mecca of learning, and were as-
sured that they would be welcomed, if they reached the hospital. In emergencies, sympathetic midwives provided
continuous emotional support to mothers who made the
drive to Andrew Memorial Hospital. Cynthia Wilson, a lifelong Tuskegee resident, captured some of the Black Belt
pride in Tuskegee when she explained that it is often said,
"When white folks die, they want to go to heaven, but when
black folks die, they want to come to Tuskegee."

## Problems with Collaboration

Midwives' feelings about local medical authorities could be
ambivalent. Mrs. Smith, who worked under the auspices of
the Greene County health department, adhered to the rules
outlined in the health department's manual for midwifery
training, but she also respected and met the needs of her patients. The rule book, for example, required Mrs. Smith to put
newborn babies in separate sleeping quarters from their
mothers—even if all they had was a cardboard box. Some
mothers preferred to keep their babies in bed with them. The
midwife safety rules stated that using any drugs other than

castor oil or another laxative to bring on labor was illegal. Some mothers wanted traditional herbs. And the rules prohibited applying any grease to the mother's abdomen or birth canal, reflecting concerns for reducing infections. Such mandates may have prevented women from receiving the age-old comfort of massage in pregnancy and labor. As health department nurses made more frequent inspections of midwifery bags for their contents, midwives prepared one bag for inspection and another for carrying to births. The bag the midwife really used might contain, in addition to legal drugs like castor oil, other oils to be mixed with sugar and turpentine for healing small cuts, and herbal roots.

Most nurses who supervised midwives did not go out on births. With the exception of public health nurses trained as nurse-midwives, supervising nurses often acquired their knowledge from lectures and textbooks and saw births only in a hospital. In 1951, when the Georgia health department hired filmmaker George Stoney to make a documentary, *All My Babies*, for training midwives, Stoney learned that public health nurses sometimes avoided going out with midwives because they feared exposing their own lack of practical experience. Nevertheless, these nurses were careful to inspect midwifery bags. Although the professional medical community labeled the use of some items found in midwifery bags as superstition, many of the old-time ways and remedies appeared to work and kept being resurrected. Many of the common postpartum rituals—salting down the afterbirth, placing open scissors under the mother's bed, and not sweeping out the ashes from the fireplace—continued long after Mrs. Smith's childbearing years.

The local physicians and nurses who respected Mrs. Smith admitted that she would make appropriate decisions in seeking referrals. Dr. Ruker Staggers, who provided backup for Mrs. Smith and delivered babies at home himself in the 1950s and 1960s, recalled, "Margaret's babies did awfully well. I can't think of any time when there was any question about Margaret's babies. But we knew that if Margaret needed us . . . there was something going on that needed some help."

While doctors valued midwives who knew when to call them, communities needed midwives who could be counted on for independent care. Before desegregation, many doctors and hospitals refused care to poor black women. Midwives resolved many complicated situations with only neighbors and friends to help out. Mrs. Smith's skill as a midwife stood up to many of the challenges she faced, allowing her, as black folks often say, to "make a way out of no way." In the course of attending thousands of women during birth, Mrs. Smith met few problems that she couldn't solve.

———

WHEN I FIRST GET TO THE MOTHER'S home, I'd see if I can find stuff to make a pad for them to deliver on. If they have some newspaper, I'd sit down and twirl that newspaper together and tack it so it won't slip and slide. If you put twenty sheets together, you won't have no trouble. See, you twirl them and fold them in a certain way, and then you tack it in each corner. I put that in the bed. That would catch the waste, so it won't get on the mattress, and it won't get on the sheet. I learned how to make the basket to catch the afterbirth out of newspaper. I learned that in Tuskegee.

Then sometimes, I'd tell the mother to go take a hot bath, and that hot water helps a lot. I sit their feet in hot water or let them sit in that tub, if they got it, a number three tub. I was willing to let them have their way until push comes to shove. Some of them would say, "I don't want to take a bath."

I'd say, "Just get in the tub, and I'll bathe you." I was right there to get them out, but some of them just wouldn't do it.

You are sitting there to do what you can for her, rub her or put something under her back, trying to rest her back some. That's what you are there for, talk to her. If you like tea, you can make them some hot tea, and that will pick them pains up. Then you can rub the stomach and make the pains start back. I'd put some grease on my hand or whatever the lady happened to have and rub it in. Sometimes I'd rub their back. That's where their misery was—in their back and stomach, but you know, if I go to rub their stomach that would make some pains rise, and they'd want me to stop rubbing their stomach, so I'd rub their back, and some of them had all their pain in their back.

Sometime they want to get up, and I'd help them up. Walk around in the room. Walk a pain off then get back in the bed. A lot of people get a kick out of walking. Go into different rooms and sit in different chairs, or get down on their knees—anywhere they think they can get ease. But there's no ease for birth till it's over with. It's good to walk, but you'll have to stop sometime. You can pretty much do what you want till you get down to the real nitty-gritty.

Now, some of the mothers be talking all this slack talk. But you're the midwife. So you, well, you got to take that. You could get up and tell them, "It doesn't make a difference. I don't care. It ain't no skin off my teeth."

I don't think that would be the words to speak. You are there. You just as well make the best out of it you can, talking kind, giving kind words and rubbing her hands. That means a lot. That means all of it. Kindness whipped the devil. Kind words, that's right, and belief. If somebody is sick, and you start talking rash to them, that hurts their feelings, but if you talk kind to them, why, that makes a lot of difference.

I'd just tell them, "Well, honey child, you're going to have to hurt before your baby's born. It ain't no way around that. You can expect that. Now the pains ain't hard now, but they're going to be hard. I want you to be aware of what's coming, and you have to learn to take it as it comes, and it will soon be over. If you are going to buck and ram and holler, you ain't going to help you none. You might as well settle yourself down and do the best you can."

See, a midwife just can't say, "You got to do so-and-so."

You know what you got to do, and you got to do it, but you can go around in a better way and make it more pleasant, the way I see it. You keep a-talking to them until they realize they got to bear to it. Some of them go to hollering when the pain comes and holler till the pain leaves, and some grunt till the pain goes off. Any way they can get an ease from that pain, they would do it, but you just keep a-talking to them until they finally make up in their mind that this is the only way. See, I've had some of them to holler till that baby gets there.

I say, "Baby, people out in the street can hear you."

They say, "I don't care if they do hear." Some of them pray, some of them moan. You got to have patience to be a midwife 'cause you got to take and give. You got to keep them entertained and in good spirits.

Let's say, if I were getting sick this morning, I would call Herlene and tell her to come up here, and she'd come and do. She'd fix my bed and do for me anything she could do. If I was hungry, she'd cook and feed me. Be right there with me. She would say, "You gonna have it—you just have to take it as it comes."

Talk consolation. That's smart things. Some people have hard long labor, and you be standing by feeling sorry for them. You would say inside of your heart, "Lord, have mercy on this person." That is very important because the Lord said to call Him pure and sincere from you heart, and He will hear you. If you're just phony, He don't go along with that. But if you say, "Lord, have mercy on this person," He really would.

One thing that makes for a long labor is when the baby be so full of dirt, white clay, sour. Eating dirt makes it hard 'cause you pushing and straining all you can with your breath, and the baby ain't moving 'cause all that stuff is gummed up on him. He can't move like he's supposed to. Now that's my idea about it. The ladies go on the highway, on these banks and things and get it. I have sent from here to Chicago to people who wanted dirt, just sent it to them, didn't charge. Women that used to live here be writing and telling me to send some dirt. So I fix them up some in a little box. Women want dirt when they're pregnant, and I sent it to them, but that was against them. I have used a big bottle of oil trying to clean this baby. It be just white, gummy, you couldn't wipe it off. Some of it, you had to leave 'cause you rupture the skin, but, Lord have mercy, it made for a hard labor.

I've had a lot of men to come in and assist me 'cause there wouldn't be anybody else there. They sit on the side of the bed, but some of the ladies wouldn't want them in there. Sometime I think that's good for the men to help, and sometime I think there are things that men should not know.

When the ladies are having hard pains, and the baby ain't showing up, making progress, I sometimes take an old shirt and put it over her—her husband's shirt. Just throw it across the shoulders, and that will help. That would get them mad, laugh, or one, and make those pains come. And I have used the man's hat. I have tried whatever people back behind me, that I have heard them say, I have tried it to see would it work, and sometime it looked like it worked, and sometime it looked like it didn't to me. That's the way I feel about it. I had learned from the older people what to do and especially Miss Ella Anderson, she taught me everything that was going to happen that did happen. She took time with me. She wanted me to go far. I think the older midwives were doing the best they could. That's the way I got it in me, in my mind.

### Kicking up Heels for Birth

See, you have a discharge that leads off in the front of the baby. Next thing will be the water breaking. Then you're getting in big business.

The time for walking is over with about near the time for the baby to be born 'cause you will see the crowning of the baby, and that's the time to quit walking. It's dangerous for the baby. It could fall, break its neck, or mash its head in. I watch it closely when the time comes, not to walk. You won't be long before you say, "Whaaaa!" You're ready then. You know that time is near. Ain't gonna stop till the baby gets here.

So those pains would pick on up. You can tell from the stomach, the way the baby is coming. If a baby is sitting up, you can tell whether the head is thisaway or you can tell whether the buttocks sit up that way or whether he's crossways.

The houses would be so cold, you would almost freeze sitting beside her bed. The fireplace up here in the front of the house, and you back over yonder on the bed. You had to peep to see what's happening down there, and you have to do it by lantern light until the people got to the place where they had better lights.

When it comes time to deliver, most of them want you to fold a quilt and put it down on the floor and turn down a straight-back chair like that one yonder with the cane-seat bottom. You put the pillows on back of it. Turn it down where they can be halfway kind of sitting up like, and their bottom part be scooted out. Somebody holds their bottom part, and somebody holds their knees. You take this chair and turn it down where she could feel the heat from the fireplace. The mother can't get cold, 'cause if she gets too cold, that's going to cut the pains down.

And then some of them get on their knees. If they're on their knees, they got some pillows on the back of the chair. They just open their knees out. Some people won't have a baby no other way but that way. Mostly there be two or three women around. They use the back of the chair to support their back, and the people help them get down.

If everything was O.K., they told us we were supposed to put the baby in a cardboard box with cotton around, but I usually put the baby in the bed with the mother.

Now a whole lot of places you go to, the afterbirth didn't come right on behind. Some of them do. Some of them don't. Sometimes the afterbirth takes twelve or thirteen hours to come loose. If you going to pull and jerk on it, you're going to leave some in there. That's going to cause a problem. If you just give it time, you work with it after the baby come. If it don't come a-loose, leave it alone. If they are tense, they need to go to sleep and relax. That makes the afterbirth come loose. Let her stretch her feet out or turn on her side or whatever she wants to do.

If the afterbirth is up in the stomach, you work with it a while. I take it and shake it and mash in the top part of the stomach. Sometime you can give it a shake and it makes the pain and zoop—right on out. Again, they may not.

I have put them over hot waters, sometimes with feathers, chicken feathers, if they want it, sometimes with nothing in it.

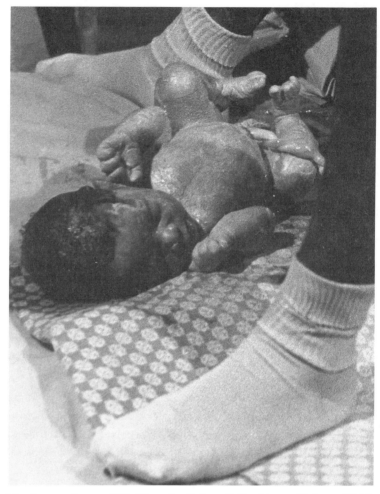

Newborn at home, 1952. Photo by Robert Galbraith, a still from *All My Babies*.

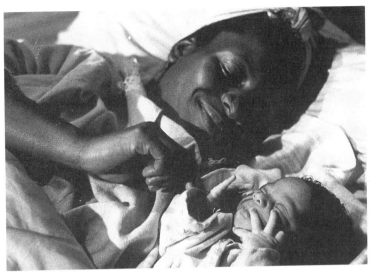

Mother and infant bonding, 1952. Photo by Robert Galbraith, a still from *All My Babies.*

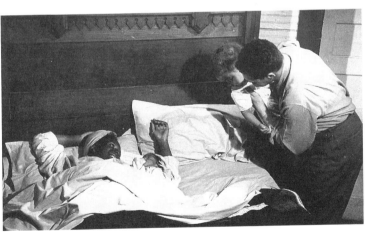

Family at birthing bed, 1952. Photo by Robert Galbraith, a still from *All My Babies.*

The old folks used to say that will make the afterbirth come loose. I've had them hang on all night, but by the next day, it turned loose.

Then I always burned my afterbirth, burned it outside the house. I burned it or made sure somebody responsible is going to burn it. We burned the afterbirth, salted it and burned it. I heard tell people burying the afterbirth. But I never did bury mine. Old folks had so many signs. Well, they always told me, Mama always said back in her day, if the dogs or something got hold of it and destroyed it, eat it up or something, you would never have another child. You say that in this day and time, people laugh at you.

At Tuskegee, we learned to take the afterbirth and turn it each way inside out and outside inside to see if any of your biscuits are missing, just like biscuits all around. If there is a piece of it left in that woman, you have to sure enough, get ready to get it out of there. Mine mostly fell out like a book.

### Tight Places

Sometimes you just be sitting there waiting for the real time to come. I remember one house, bless your soul, it was a sight. A pig was over in the corner, and a goat was over in the other corner, and I was sitting on a nail can. When I come out, I had a black circle on round where I was sitting. Her mama and daddy in one bed. She in another bed, trying to have the baby.

I said, "Uh-uh."

Wasn't a blessed thing there. Wasn't nothing there. It made you want to puke. The mother didn't have anything, I think she had seven children. They were just poor people. It didn't make no difference, you were colored anyway. That's right.

They didn't care what happened. One day, you'll die, hire another one, just didn't make no difference. It was just, just one of those things.

The best thing about the job is when you don't have to be away from home so long. Let's say you leave that morning at five o'clock and the baby comes around ten o'clock, by eleven-thirty or twelve o'clock. You're going to stay there till she comes to, then you're ready to come home. That's the best part. The baby's O.K. and the mama's O.K. But you'd get in so many places where you just can't leave.

I had to sit down there in Furse Quarters, I think it was. This is right here in Eutaw. They had a green slab board for fire, and instead of it burning, it just kept smoking.

I still figured they just could have done better. A big bar of soap only costs ten cents. You used to could wash an army of clothes off of that bar of soap. You rub them, put them in cold water, rub them again, get as much dirt out of them as you can, rub the soap off them, drop them in the pot, and let them boil. Then take your stick and work them 'round, take them out of there and rub them again, put them in that rinse water. If you had bluing, put a drop or two in your white clothes before hanging them up. Then people used to make soap. Mama made a many of jar full, but people just quit doing anything. They could have had at least a clean sheet, a clean quilt. I had to go next door just for rags. I always figured that big fish swallowed the little one. The white folks had the colored under control. We were living in slavery, and white folks didn't care.

So, that next evening, here I was still sitting there. When morning come, I went to Randolph's cousin's house to get something to eat or coffee. I looked like a dog.

I said, "I ain't fit to come in."

I stayed on the porch and drank that coffee. It was good,

too, and as soon as I drank the coffee, back it come. I threw every bit back, but I got me a dip of snuff, and went on. You got to be strong and tough.

A wagon, a one-horse wagonman came and got me from the Quarters. I couldn't stand it. I was weak. Soon as I got home, I got buck naked on the back porch, in broad daylight, naked, and tipped on back in the house. I said, many more nights like this, and I'm putting this midwife work down.

The nurse would come after the baby was born, if I gave her word to come. If you weighed the baby, and the baby is underweight, then you call your nurse to bring out the incubator. They used to have the one that runs with hot water bottles.

I'd always try to go back after the third day. Most of them, you tell them to get up every morning and wash off, but they wouldn't do it. They definitely weren't getting into a tub of water. No use saying that 'cause they weren't going to do it. They believed it would kill them if they did that. They weren't going to do it, uh-uh. Don't let the mother get cold. Like this fan here, you couldn't sit under this fan. You couldn't open that door. They say you catch cold. Back then, they didn't wash their hair in six months. Now they wash their hair any time they get ready. Well, they give you that for a reason, they say, but what reason I don't know.

I had a lady had the door just cracked, and here it was so hot in that house. It was in September. We used to say, if the baby's born at home, you got to keep the fire burning one night, twelve hours, then it can go out. You couldn't take a fire out of the fireplace where the mother was for four or five days.

The midwife would slip a knife, sharp fork, or scissors under the bed, between the bed and the mattress, but you didn't have to let the person know it was there. You had to put it in there the day after, when they were asleep. Open the scissors and point them down or point them up. That helps ease the pain. In her [the mother's] absence, just catch her. Like I'm tucking in the sheet and just stick those scissors under there and let them be open, and it helps a whole lot. It soothes those pains down.

One while, there was nobody that was going to nurse a baby. Back in them days, they'd take needles and string them and let them hit right down between your breasts and that would let their milk out. Pour the milk out on a hot brick until it dries up. I put three or four sewing needles, many as I could find, not over four or five and just thread them and hang them down between their bosom.

But, if you wanted to nurse, just take a comb and comb that breast down. A hair comb breaks it like you do a cow bag. Yeah, break them clots, like holding the calf when you milk her, first time you milk her, feel it come down in the titties.

### Ban on Teas

Now, the nurses didn't know what was good and what was bad. You can take too much of anything. You just need enough to warm you up inside and get those pains a-moving, if you done done everything you can do on the outside.

I had to stop fooling with teas and things in labor because my name was getting out.

"Miss Margaret, how come you are not using some of that stuff you used on Emma or Lucille. She was telling me about what good stuff you had. Why don't you give me some? Fix some for me so I can get through with this baby."

See, my name was getting where I could hear it. I stopped right then. I had been practicing a good while. I was going by what Miss Ella Anderson taught, but I stopped. I already knew about the teas 'cause I was going with this other midwife. They used to make teas for the mothers to pick the pains up.

The woman told us in the clinic, I think we had a meeting of all the midwives, the woman was from Selma.

She said, "No more pepper tea, no dirt dauber, no kind of root or nothing unless you give them some hot tea, regular. But not no roots and things like that."

They said, "They better not catch nobody giving nobody no tea of no kind. If they do, she was going to jail and from there to the pen."

So, I didn't figure I wanted to go to the pen, but they had a couple midwives that still gave a woman teas. They had the nurses to come and the doctor that was the head of the clinic, and a couple more white ladies. I don't know who they were or where they were from. But they sure got that midwife ripped about them teas. They told her the best thing you do when you go home, get your bag and come back to town. Bring your bag in because you're going to kill somebody.

You know, they're quick to think teas and things are going to kill somebody. One midwife told the nurse when we had the meeting, she just told her, "I think I'll bring my bag in and give it to you all because you all are not there when this labor is going on. You don't know how it goes. Rubbing helps and teas help. If I can't give them some hot teas which I know will help, I just well ought to give it up."

And I felt like this about it. Various people, if you do something to help them, when they get up on their feet, they're going to tell somebody, and it keeps going 'round till it works back to the white folks, and there you go. They're going to know what you're doing or how much you're doing or where you're doing it at. I cut off because I was grown enough and old enough to know what people would do, just like they

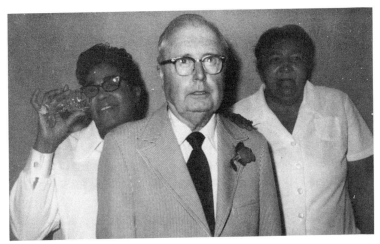

Joshie Lee McCoy (LPN, clinic aide), Dr. Sidney Williams, and Margaret Charles Smith at the health department, Eutaw, mid-1960s. Photo courtesy of Margaret Charles Smith.

doing in this day and time, they going to get in your business. I figured I done took the oath, and I'm going to work on anyhow till the end.

I told Hattie right down at the clinic, "I'm through with them teas. They're just going to have those babies with what the guide says, 'cause they told us not to try to help them."

So I quit. I quit trying to do anything but what they gave me to work with. I had been working a good while when I threw that root out my bag.

## Surviving Complications

A midwife has a thousand-dollar responsibility on her. If you had somebody to come in, a doctor or somebody, they could lighten the burden on you. But as long as I got to be there to see what the outcome will be, whatever it is, I got to report it. You have to go through it, the good and the bad. A midwife goes through with more than the doctor goes through with.

You really got to know. It takes somebody who knows how to get up and make a move and try to get the mother somewhere. Her blood pressure may be up or she may be threatening to have convulsions, chewing her tongue up. If she gets to doing that, you have to wrap a spoon or board and stick it in her mouth to keep her from eating her tongue up. You got a lot of responsibility on your hands.

It's a sin, because the midwife has all the brunt to bear on her. If anything happens bad to the mother, they're calling you in. The doctor goes there and does what he's going to do. Gives her a shot and bye-bye. It may do good or it won't do good, bye-bye.

The underground is you working, you deliver the baby, but you aren't supposed to be there. You don't have a license to be there. See, they never did allow the midwives to deliver white people. But I did. When I go to deliver the baby, if this lady has been to the doctor, all I had to do was carry that birth certificate to the doctor, and I'm through with it. They could sign it for me. That's the reason I say you got to have somebody to stand behind you what in ever happens, death or whatever happens. You got to have somebody that knows, that's been seeing this person, then you got somebody. If you go there barehanded, and they ask what doctor have you been to or what clinic you've been to, you got a doctor to call.

I delivered the head nurse at our clinic. She was white, and I'd just started the midwife work. We could nurse the white people, but they never did allow the midwives to deliver white people. She fixed everything up well, padded her bed, got the clothes out, the pan for water, and walked around before she decided to sit down. She just really wanted me there to catch the baby. She showed me where to cut the cord, and that's what I did, just like she told me, yes ma'am.

Then she got up and started cooking. She wasn't from around here, no way. But there was plenty of poor white people who was just like the poor colored people. They didn't have nothing. But this nurse, she just wanted me, wanted me to be with her. I stayed with her four nights and four days. She just wanted me.

## Segregated Health Systems

One time, I had twins, and the woman had high blood pressure. She was diabetic. The doctor always told me when they was going to be twins, but he didn't tell me about them two. Before I knew anything here comes the second baby. So the mother was awfully weak. She had seven children before she had the twins, and the fact of the business was, she worked hard anyway.

After the last baby came, we called the doctor. All right, I got both of the babies. But just as fast as I can get her to come to with alcohol, camphor, and stuff, she went out again. I told her husband, "Look, you get out from here. Call the doctor."

She had a doctor, but we were a long ways. I said, "He saw her all through her pregnancy. You tell him to come and come quick. This woman has a high blood and sugar. She's bleeding too much. The more I surgery her, the more blood comes, and she passes out."

I tried everything in the book. I even had salt in the middle of her head with alcohol. I had a rag so it wouldn't run down in her eye. She had a quilt in between her legs. We were just wringing the blood out. I kept trying to massage her stomach to stop the bleeding.

When he came, the doctor said to me, "Margaret, what's the matter?"

I 'called myself wanting to explain to him what the trouble was as far as I knew.

He said, "I'll tell you what you ought to have done. You ought to have got a bucket of water and poured it on her." Now those are the words he gave me.

I said, "Well, I'll tell you, I left that for you to do." I was looking at him dead in his face. I was getting mad then.

He gave her one shot in her arm and reached down and got his little grip, out the door. I said, "Lord have mercy. If this woman here dies on me, wooh."

That shot didn't raise her a bit, uh-uh. It was in my mind, if she doesn't stop bleeding soon, I'd have to carry her to the hospital. I kept trying to massage her stomach till I could get it hard like a grapefruit to stop the bleeding. But as soon as I get it hard, it quits, and here comes the blood.

See, most of the doctors weren't too lovely with the colored folk. They had to make their money. That's the only reason they had to try to go along with them, but I had to sit there all day long, and she was regularly a-passing out. I was there from midnight until twelve o'clock the next day. And that lady is still living right now.

A lot of hospitals around here, they just wouldn't fool with you. The only place we had to carry a patient to was Tuskegee, and that was a long ways from here. I've carried about four or five to Tuskegee. I carried one girl with TB. That was a good bit of travel.

Now some of the ladies went to Tuskegee to get their tubes tied. You know, they had a complaint, anything irregular, doctor didn't want to fool with them any more with the condition they were in. They'd go over to Tuskegee. Lots of them had so many babies they were worn completely out.

I don't know how much they charged them to get to Tuskegee, but you had eight months to make a reservation to get somebody to take you, and some of them set on their butts the whole nine months. But them that went with the health center, we carried them free.

## An Emergency Case

Another girl, Mary Harris, she lives in this first brick house on the right, she was born in my lap. That's right, right downtown, heart of Montgomery, born in my lap. We had a good piece to go from here to Tuskegee. I was just as bloody as if somebody had cut me up in pieces. She [the mother] was having convulsions and the doctor said he wouldn't take a chance on it, so he called himself giving her a shot to hold her pains down until we got there.

I was right down to the traffic light in Montgomery, stopped, and here comes the baby, nowhere else to be born but in my lap. I was just as bloody as a hog. I had to take my hand and pull her up and lay her on my leg, and the old piece of quilt that her mama put in the car, I pulled it up over her back, and that's the way we rode to Tuskegee, her legs just shaking. The mother, she bled like a cow. Her legs and everything, just shaking, and I just looked like I was cut up in pieces.

I reckon the reason why she continued to have those convulsions was her afterbirth didn't come. If she had of been born in all that litter, and her face had of been turned down or either if she had her mouth open, she could have been gone.

The nurse, she was driving. She stopped the highway patrol and asked them to open the road 'cause she had an emergency case. He got in front of us, and you talk about flying! I said, "God, they're going to kill us all."

We got to Tuskegee, but I was just in no shape to go in. I was in one mess. I was mad about the nurse asking me about going in with me looking the way I was. I looked like I was cut up in pieces. I was wet, too. The water had done broken. So I stayed in the car till the nurse was ready to go back to Eutaw.

The mother stayed, and the baby stayed in Tuskegee, but we come back to Eutaw that night. The mother continued having convulsions after the baby came. She was having them when we left Eutaw, and she had them when she got in the hospital.

That blood never did come out of my dress. It always looked yellow, don't care what I did to that white uniform. I soaked that uniform when I got home, and I put Clorox on everything down to my drawers, and that didn't do any good. They had to get a new seat on the car to clean it out. I knew they had a job, but I was in a worse shape. That gal thinks well of me now 'cause I saved her life, bless her soul, she's as sweet as anything. When I was sick, she always called asking about me, and she sent me a basket of fruit.

### More Problems

I've had plenty of them with the cord around the neck. When the baby's head come out, you automatically see the cord. When the mother has a pain, you used to put your finger in there and slip or loop it, loop it over, bring it over his head. Sometimes it will be wrapped three or four times. As long as the cord is wrapped around there, it's kind of choking like, pulling. The baby can't get the air to breathe like it should 'cause that cord is caught around its neck. I've done it so many times. I didn't need a doctor for that.

Sometimes I had to break the bag of water. I break it when I see the bag. I have a stick, you know, with a sharp point—a toothpick or something—and I stick it. When it's hanging off from the baby's head, you break it. But you don't break it up in the vagina. You let it come out some before you stick it.

Then I've had them come foot first. I didn't have much luck turning them. That's the way they coming, they coming that way. I always had to push one foot back and get both feet together 'cause ain't nothing going to happen with one foot coming out first. You push that one foot back and get both of the feet, and let both of the feet come down together. And then some time the hands would be up over their little heads, and you have to put on a glove and go up in there and get an arm and bring it down before they can pass through.

I had a breech baby up here in Mantua. Everything was fine. Next time I looked there was that foot, sticking out there.

I said, "Oh, my goodness. We taking you to the doctor right now."

Sure enough we didn't try to change clothes or nothing, just put her in the car and carried her on to the city and just did make it there five minutes before time.

And then, it's all right to deliver a baby weighing six or seven pounds, seven and a half or something like that, and it come breech baby, but now, if it weighed eight, nine, ten pounds, you gonna have a scuffle to get that baby out in time. Well, when you find out it has a foot coming first, you know it's going to be a breech baby when you see those little toes. And you better get away from there before he come on out, till he get to up there to them shoulders. There's your problem, right across them shoulders, and you got to whirl it. If you don't, you got a dead baby. In five minutes you got to have that baby out. I was able to, you know, the Lord didn't let me have but one, and she was so big. And when I got there the baby's whole foot and things were out, and I said, "Call the doctor."

The mother down on her knees, and the baby was regularly coming. I said, "Ain't nobody you can send to tell the doctor?" Wasn't no phones to tell the doctor to come here quick. I said, "Well, I'll be darned."

That was a big baby, and she was diabetic too, and them babies be big. See, everything's all right until you get along here with them shoulders, then you gonna work there to get that baby turned to get out of there. Yes, sir. You got to get those shoulders out and head out, too.

Then sometimes, they couldn't bear no more. They were tired and worried about pain. You supposed to been bearing to it to help push the baby on down. You better know what you doing when you fooling with folks that are diabetic. You better let them go 'head, because the baby be too big. Any doctor will tell you that. Somebody's got to go a mile before you get some help—but those five minutes after you get the bottom part of the baby out—you got to work. You got five minutes to get this baby out! Pheew! You got to put your gloves on to turn that baby. You turn him on one of his shoulders and let him slide on out till he get to the head. Now suppose she don't bear. There he is. You got to go in there and help that baby, 'cause it gets to the place where she won't bear no more. There you are again, whoo! That's too much a go for me.

When it leaves that neck part, you got to put your hands under that baby's neck back there and go as far as you can go helping him on, to get him out. That's the dangerous part. That's the reason why if I see a foot, just as much as them toes, I'm getting away from there before the next thing comes, 'cause it ain't going to be long before I need some help. I been in some tough spots, I tell you.

Another bad birth is butt backwards. You know the butt part comes out first. You got some trouble on your hands. You got to sure 'nough work to get it out. But it so happened the Lord didn't let them be too long before they come on through. It takes a pretty good while because it is doubled up under the butt, the little feet were doubled up under him.

You don't turn it. You just get to moving when those feet get down low enough, you get that foot and bring it down and go back up in there and get that other foot and bring it down and that will give the baby room to come on down till you get up there to them shoulders. Then you got to get a lean. If there's enough room, you don't have to do nothing else. It will come right on. Then sometimes again it won't, but you got to sure know when and where so you'll know what to do. It's a sight.

Now I never cut them. They always bust. Then they had to get them sewed up. Now some doctors split it [did an episiotomy], and then the baby come on. I said, nope. Sometimes they just split wide open and that lets the baby come on out there.

But if she just gets a small tear when she's having that baby, something like a skin burst, but not tearing in the flesh, I just put a little sugar, and a little grease, vaseline—pure vaseline on her pad—turpentine too, and she'll do nicely.

See, if she bust, I always carried them and let somebody stitch 'em up. See, you can tell when the water break, you can tell how well the head is proceeding, 'cause there is room down in there to feel the head. And while she bearing, you can feel the head slipping and so, you got to just sit there and wait.

But if the head ain't moving, you in trouble still. I'll see how much she done dilated. See if the baby is crowning, and that means the head is coming out, but if you don't see that head, you better get away. Somebody better move, 'cause you in trouble. And another dangerous thing is the afterbirth can separate from the baby. It can come first. That's dangerous, real dangerous.

A black lady here used to stick that womb to make the baby come before time. I delivered one where the baby came out in pieces. I had to pick that baby out piece by piece. She did something to try to destroy the baby, and I had this cardboard box putting the pieces in. But you know, some people got hurt, scratches. It's hard to cure, especially being diabetic, and some of them are hard to cure regardless of what.

I used to make up alum and white of egg and some quinine, little quinine and make a balm, what you call a balm for female trouble. It is a big roll of cotton, and tie a good string on it good. That's for when their womb is down. They feel lots better in a couple of days. They'd be all right. Had to put a drop of turpentine in it.

## Medical Compromises

Another time I was up and down the road all night with this lady 'cause the doctor, he wouldn't come out there. After the baby was born, I'm so sharp, I'm just as sharp as he is. I took the mother and the baby into his office. Wrapped the baby up and got an old quilt and wrapped her up, and then he didn't want to see her. She had a high blood, sure enough.

See, if I get there and see it's coming the wrong way, I have to get out there and carry her to the hospital, the doctor, or one. When we got to the doctor, I said, "Now aren't you going to give her something? I brought her to you because she's bleeding so bad. I thought you would do something for her."

He said, "Yeah, but she had plenty time. She had nine

months to get ready for this baby, but she didn't do nothing, and what is she doing now, nothing."

I said, "Well, probably wasn't nothing she could do. What could she do, but suffer with high blood? Wasn't too much she could do."

That's me.

He said, "She wouldn't eat right. She wouldn't do right. This kind of case just aggravates you to death."

He just preached to a funeral. He preached so long you could have gone across the water on a ship. He said, "Her husband could have gone to his boss man, if he needed a way to get to the hospital."

The doctor knew she didn't have money to go to Demopolis, a hospital. She didn't have nothing to go to Tuscaloosa or Tuskegee. She didn't have nothing to pay the man who drove her to the doctor that night. She didn't have a dollar.

I do believe that the only thing that made him give her a shot was when I told him that something had to be done. It happened, and something had to be done.

That man that drove us to the doctor, he was out there on the road grumbling about his money. He said his car was messed up, and it was. I took my money out of my pocket and paid him to come get her and carry her to the doctor, 'cause I was afraid she might die.

I said, "Lord, I can get in some of the worse mess there ever was."


## Premature Baby

I had one baby weighed two and a half pounds. Know what I had to do? I had to get some whiskey bottles and heat me some water and wrap it, wrapped them whiskey bottles with the hot water and put a towel around it, and then put the bottles all around the baby. Had but three bottles, one for the head, the side, and the one at the foot to keep heat until I could get an incubator. They had them running then, not by electricity.

I had to do this with a girl in school who got pregnant. See, they didn't allow you in school. If you were pregnant, you had to come out. So this girl didn't want nobody to know she was pregnant. She got a plain sack, like yellow domestic, folded that thing, and she got somebody to fix her up with safety pins, real nice and neat. She wore that till she had the baby. She went to school that evening and had the baby that night. It was in March, and I had to cut the sack off of her before she had the baby to give the baby a chance. Then I had to get those whiskey bottles to keep the baby warm.

It's a trip. It ain't as easy as folk think it is. Worth every dime you made, and folks promise to pay you and won't pay. I said, "Lord, have mercy, if I had just had money that folks owed me."

# | 5 |

# CIVIL RIGHTS

*By the 1950s, the mood* in Alabama had changed radically as the movement for civil rights exploded. In 1954 the U.S. Supreme Court had declared, in *Brown v. Board of Education of Topeka, Kansas,* that "separate but equal" had no place in public education. In 1955 a 381-day bus boycott in Montgomery was set off by Rosa Parks's arrest for refusing to go to the back of the bus. The year 1957 saw passage of the Civil Rights Act, a mechanism for challenging local registrars denying blacks the vote. The long and ardent march to justice peaked in Alabama's racial confrontations of the 1960s, which included murders of both white and black civil rights workers, attacks on demonstrators with hoses and dogs, and the brutal Birmingham killing of black children in a Sunday school bombing.

Official state leadership upheld the status quo through law, police power and violence, and intimidation and crackdowns on activists. It tried to mold public opinion through the conservative media. Local newspapers provided information on black political action—but only to illustrate how racial equality could never become a reality. Early congressional pleas to dismantle segregation and quell racial violence fell on deaf ears. In a March 4, 1948, article in the *Greene County Democrat,* for example, Frank P. Samford, president of Alabama's Chamber of Commerce, condemned emerging congressional civil rights proposals to repeal the poll tax, make lynching a federal offense, and abolish segregation of the races as a blow to states' rights.

In 1955 the twenty-nine-year-old Rev. Ralph T. Abernathy, a native of Alabama's Marengo County and pastor of a Montgomery church, described the appalling socioeconomic conditions. Abernathy's complaints about lack of resources—including medical care—and his descriptions of the difficulties blacks faced in obtaining access to services echoed Booker T. Washington's laments from the 1890s:

> The mid-1950's life was most difficult for all poor people, but it was much better for poor white people than for black people in the South. Blacks were permitted to hold only the menial jobs, domestic workers and common and ordinary laborers. The only professional jobs that were open to blacks were the field of pastoring a black church and the school teaching profession, which was open because of segregated schools. Whites didn't normally teach black students. In the whole state of Alabama we had probably less than five black doctors. And we didn't do anything but dig ditches and work with some white supervisor that told us everything to do. We were the last to be hired and the first to be fired. (Quoted in Hampton, 18–19)

Although civil rights activism challenged inequities in schools, public facilities, and employment with some success, barriers to comprehensive medical care remained. Between 1955 and 1964, little progress was made statewide in improving infant mortality rates. Statistics from the state health department show that nonwhite infant mortality was actually higher in 1964 than in 1955. Even though the number of black out-of-hospital births dropped dramatically, there was no significant downward trend in infant mortality rates in the 1950s or 1960s. A study of out-of-hospital deliveries between 1940 and 1980 reported that more than 90 percent of all black babies were born out of hospital in 1940, compared to 46 percent in 1960. In 1964, a study of infant mortality in Alabama put the white infant mortality rate at 23.2 per 1,000, or slightly lower than the national average. The black infant mortality rate was nearly twice that, and significantly higher than the national average.

An investigation conducted by the Tuskegee Institute School of Nursing and supported by a Public Health Services Research Grant documented the continued dependency of rural blacks on the Andrew Memorial Hospital for care of premature infants. The hospital admitted more babies between 1961 and 1965, a five-year period, than it did during the fifteen-year period between 1951 and 1965. According to the *Final Report of the Effect of Nursing Care on Selected Aspects of Premature Infant Welfare in the Home,* black mothers and babies from forty-two of Alabama's sixty-seven counties still came to Andrew Memorial Hospital because, as the report concluded, "Several of these 42 counties have no hospital while those with hospitals are in most instances reluctant to admit indigent Negro mothers and their premature infants. For this and other reasons, a significant number of mothers of premature infants who can afford the travel expenses are referred or come to John A. Andrew Memorial Hospital" (6).

Greene County opened its first public hospital in 1966. Although constructed with federal Hill-Burton funds, this facility continued to practice illegal segregation even after the signs were removed. James Coleman, the executive director of Greene County's first comprehensive health clinic (opened 1974), recalled "going over to the hospital in 1969–70, and one day there were two waiting rooms. The next day they closed one because an inspector was coming, but nothing really changed." Dr. Joe Bethany, a Greene County native

115

who set up his Eutaw medical practice in 1960, remembered, "When I built this office, I built two waiting rooms because that was the way it was done. When this became a major issue, we just took the signs down, and then people continued pretty much to segregate themselves like that." Even in the 1970s and early 1980s, the private offices of some Greene County physicians remained segregated and were staffed only by whites.

## Struggles for Change

Eutaw, which epitomized much of the Old South, proudly anchored itself in the past. During the era of civil rights demonstrations, Bill Lee, the county sheriff (who had been captain of the Alabama University football team and had played professionally for the Green Bay Packers) boasted that he did not need a gun to maintain law and order in Greene County: His reputation carried enough power. In the early 1960s, Mrs. Smith recalls walking down the main street of Eutaw and seeing the worst of the Eutaw retaliation against activists. She said, "They killed one boy right here on the street. It was some rough stuff when they were beating people up." She also saw the sheriff kick a woman in the stomach near Eutaw's drugstore. Although Mrs. Smith was not directly involved in the movement, her oldest son, Houston, did speak out locally against racial inequality.

Mrs. Smith was working at the maternity clinic in Tishibe, less than twenty miles from Eutaw, when civil rights workers marched down the road in front of the clinic. She said, "They'd put a bullet in your butt. It was rough down there in Tishibe." George Perry, who now lives in Forkland, Greene County, recalls his own activism, which included marches in Tishibe:

White people were mad because the black people were
marching out there. I wasn't scared, 'cause when you
get started in that movement, you weren't scared. If
you trust in the Lord, you don't be worried about what
happened. And God took care of me. Nobody but God
took care of us. . . .

Black people were treated so bad. People treated so
bad, boy. Take our women. Do all that stuff to black
folks. Take a man's wife and go home and go to bed
with them. Man standing right out in the field and they
didn't do nothing. They scared. It was rough. Take a
man's wife and carry her home and the man standing
right up there. It was rough. Man out there in the field
and take his wife home. Enough to make you cry.

Mrs. Smith speaks openly about her decades of work under
whites before the civil rights movement. She recalls, "I
worked like a dog, but white folks didn't love you. You
couldn't eat in the cafes. If you did, you had to go to the back.
Before civil rights, I rode to Bessemer [about seventy miles
from Eutaw] standing up all the way because the seats were
in the front for white people only."

The civil rights era signaled some changes for midwives.
Before it, Mrs. Smith had helped an interracial couple expecting a baby because they feared the response of a white doctor. When Mrs. Smith cared for white women, she usually
had a white doctor sign the birth certificate. Herlene Pipping
agrees that the civil rights movement changed clandestine
practices. According to her, "Before Martin Luther King
came through, they did a lot of things under cover. If a white
person did use a black midwife at that time, they would
hardly want anyone to know that she's the one who did it."

A film about Greene County, *Time and Dreams*, on de-
posit at the Museum of Modern Art film library in New York,

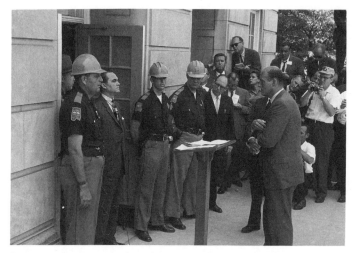

Governor Wallace blocking the entrance to the University of Alabama, Tuscaloosa, 1963. Photo by Warren K. Lessler. Library of Congress Prints, *U.S. News and World Report.*

shows the reluctance of some Eutaw whites to yield to changing times for years after the ardent civil rights struggles. Ten years after Governor George Wallace took his infamous 1955 stance in the door of the University of Alabama, Greene County school children feared for their safety under court-ordered school desegregation. One newspaper reported that Governor Wallace issued a restraining order forbidding Martin Luther King Jr. from participating in any marches in Greene County in 1967. Local demonstrations demanded more police protection for blacks wishing to transfer their children to previously segregated schools. One of Eutaw's black mothers filed a federal suit against state troopers, charging them with keeping her daughter from entering school grounds. Meanwhile, local whites opened an all-white private high school, Warrior Academy, to avoid complying with school desegregation orders. Racism was so entrenched in Greene County that Ralph Abernathy grabbed Tuscaloosa headlines in 1969 when he said that winning the right to vote in Greene County was more historic than man's walk on the moon.

The civil rights movement revolutionized the political structure of Greene County. In 1969, it became the first place in the country to have blacks assume political power in the county government. The intense organizing, struggle, and sacrifice following passage of the Voting Rights Act had finally borne fruit. A slate made up mostly of local farmers became the first black county commission. The old courthouse, site of white vigilantism during Reconstruction and a Ku Klux Klan rallying point in the mid-1960s, was rebaptized when a mostly black crowd of more than a thousand people—some in Sunday frocks and others in African garb—gathered to celebrate election-day victories. That same day, a parade led by Abernathy spilled into a spontaneous liberation swim in Eutaw's still segregated, all-white swimming pool. Then in 1970, Alabama's first black probate judge since Reconstruction, William McKinley Branch, a former teacher and a preacher, was voted into the most powerful elective office in Greene County, and Thomas Earl Gilmore, also a black man, was appointed sheriff. Collectively these victories signaled that political change had come: 103 southern counties followed Greene County in electing black candidates for the first time since Reconstruction. Many believed that the biblical prophecy of the last being first was coming true in this life.

The political gains made during the movement began slipping away in the Reagan-Bush era. Eutaw's Dr. Joe P. Smith, for example, worked diligently to woo black voters away from their former political power base. Local blacks accused him of threatening to deny them health care if they did

119

not follow his political preferences. Meanwhile local whites leveled allegations of voting fraud against black politicians.

## Long-Lasting Barriers

Improving services and overturning the effects of decades of nonrepresentation presented challenges that outlived any political celebration. Although federal dollars began to flow into Greene County, augmenting the funds available for housing, health, and other social services, the problem of poverty remained. Greene County was one of the poorest counties in the state and, indeed, in the nation. According to a report from the U.S. Commission on Civil Rights, Greene County in 1970 had the highest percentage of families living below the poverty level of any county in Alabama. In that year, the median income for blacks was $2,280. The local cattle, timber, and cotton industries could not support all those who needed work, and most of the few jobs open to local blacks paid poorly. In the 1970s, a franchise for a dog-racing park with parimutuel betting was awarded to a group headed by Tuscaloosa's Paul Bryant Jr., son of Alabama football coach Paul "Bear" Bryant. The park brought in some additional tax revenues for the county, but it fell short of expectations in the number of full-time jobs it created.

Mrs. Smith knows too well the realities of racial and social injustices, and she has never lost her fear of white violence. Once, however, Mrs. Smith took advantage of her relationship with a white employer and asked for her assistance in crossing a civil rights picket line. In Eutaw, as in other towns across Alabama and the South, many of those on the picket line were younger than Mrs. Smith. Her complex political consciousness has been shaped as much by the whites who have been a part of her life in Greene County as by young blacks afire with new political zeal. Times remained hard for many in Greene County, despite the political changes made possible by the civil rights movement.

And hard times continued for Mrs. Smith. As the number of births she attended declined by the mid-1970s, she was forced to accept more work as a live-in nurse, taking care of white infants in their homes. Although jobs like nursing paid better than midwifery, it meant assuming the submissive behavior of a domestic worker.

---

THERE BE ABOUT TWO HUNDRED PEOPLE commenced to marching right here in Eutaw. They would go all around just singing and clapping. Some people lost their lives for it. Some people got kicked in the butt. Those folks, white folks, would be peeping to see who that was on their plantation. You're going to get a letter day after that, you had to go, had to move.

They burned down the houses. They took the tops off, tin roofs, burned the houses down, if they found out you were in that march. Now my cousin down here, her son went to Tishibe, and a van pulled up with boys and things. What happened? When the news come, he was dead.

See, the folks be marching every day, and the white people didn't like that. The white people would stand out and see who was in this march, and after that, next week or so they get a letter. They have to move. White folks be out there looking to see who was in that march so they could write them a letter. To keep anybody from getting the house, they tear that house down. Tough. Tough here in Eutaw.

But still they marched. They marched till they closed them stores up and made them take half that stuff to the dump. Sure

# K.K.K.
# RALLY

## Sunday, October 24, 1965
## 2:30 P.M.
## Eutaw Alabama

### Whites Cordially Invited

To Hear -

Robert Shelton, Imperial Wizard
Bob Creel, Grand Dragon of Alabama
and others

Sponsored by: United Klans Of America
Charter No. 47, Eutaw, Ala.

United Klan announcement, 1965, *Greene County Democrat.*

the march, and they'd have a smart remark to make about, "I ain't gonna let you have nothing else, you needn't come to me for nothing else."

That didn't make no difference. They closed the stores up. That's right. All that stuff—they had to haul it to the dump. My oldest son, he knew what was right and what was wrong, 'cause sometime he spoke down there at the courthouse, and I'd be so scared I didn't know what to do. I'd be scared he wasn't going to make it home. They had a meeting at the courthouse every so often on a Sunday night or Wednesday night. I begged him to stay home. I didn't want nobody to hurt him.

He said, "This was a free country. I've been over to Vietnam and over some of everywhere. I lost my health, and I'm going come home and I ain't free?"

I didn't want to go the marches. I just didn't feel like I wanted to go, 'cause I didn't want nobody hitting on me or kicking on me for nothing, 'cause I haven't done nothing. That's the way I felt about it. I just didn't want to be in it, 'cause white folks going to kick me—uh-uh-uh-uh. 'Cause I might have been marching for better.

I saw Martin Luther King. I was close to him, where they stopped the limousine, right down here in Eutaw. He made a speech from there, and he circled on around town and went back to the schoolhouse or church or somewhere. I thought he was great. Then after the white folks got to treating the colored folks so bad I said oowee! These white folks tough here now!

The first year they started, they caught me in the A & P. At that time, my husband was living. They never bothered me, but I had a husband who had his leg amputated up to his knees. I had to go to the A & P, and I told them, "I have to go somewhere. I have one husband. He can't walk. I got a husband in a wheelchair with one leg. He has to have a certain kind of food that I can't find anywhere else but Tuscaloosa or Aliceville."

He was crazy about sweetening, diet peaches, and that's what caused me to go in the A & P, 'cause they were the only people who carried that kind of stuff. They told me to go to Tuscaloosa or somewhere else.

I said, "I'm sorry, but I'm going to have to go in there. I've done worked like a dog all day, and I'm going to take my money to buy the food for transportation. I won't have any money to buy the food with, if I have to pay for somebody to carry me to the grocery shop. He has a certain kind of food that I can't find any other place than the A & P."

She said, "You send by somebody."

Now, it costs six dollars to get a car to go to Aliceville. And I'm supposed to go way over there and my husband is down sick. You know that was wrong. Somebody has somebody sick in their house, and they can't really work for themselves. I got to do it all and try to work too. I can't do all these things. They threatened me, but I went on in. I had to. I was the only somebody to look out for my husband, and I had to go to the A & P to get this food, but I got scared.

So I got the white lady I was working for to go and get me different things. I thanked her, yes ma'am, 'cause it saved me.

### Old Hunting Club

The clinic, a club it used to be, that's what we had for a clinic, a log cabin where the hunters used to meet. The school buses come in. I believe it was about six or seven buses, and commenced to parking all the way around, and they started singing that we'll overcome.

We were carrying on clinic, dressing the ladies and putting them up, and the doctor was there. The doctor could hear them, and everybody else could, too. The doctor got so mad he couldn't say nothing. He didn't say nothing to me. He didn't say nothing to nobody. The doctor didn't open his mouth, he was so mad.

I had to go out there and tell the people that were in their gowns to put back on their clothes 'cause the doctor wasn't going to see them. He was so mad, shit. He didn't know what to do. The doctor threw that specimen down. He pulled the gloves off and threw them down. When the doctor threw his gloves down, I picked them up and put them in a box to bring them back to Eutaw. That was my job.

124

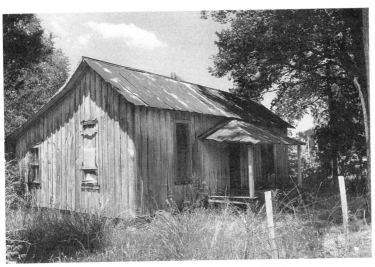
Old Tishibe clinic, 1995. Photo by Sharon Blackmon.

It was just a jam. It was tough. I felt sorry for some of the ladies, because they had a hard way to get about. There was so many people coming to the clinic. It be loaded out, stuffed up with people.

The march come through because people wanted them to have better clinics that were open more days during the week. They came down one Thursday and closed the clinic down. Made the doctor mad, and he left. Made the nurse mad, and she left.

They closed it up from that day on. Left the patients lying on the table with their legs up in the air. That caused the ladies to have nowhere to go unless they went to Demopolis to a doctor. They had to pay there.

Tishibe is a big place, and sometimes the ladies be late getting there, and the nurse done closed the books—the part that she's supposed to do before the doctor comes, like checking their blood pressure, taking their blood, and checking urine.

125

The nurse be done and closed that part when the lady comes walking up and say she didn't have a way. A lot of them had to get out, walk part the way to catch a way.

That day we came back to Eutaw, me and the nurse, and she cried all the way from Tishibe to Eutaw. Her dress was wet from crying. She didn't take time to get no paper towels. Her face looked like blood was going to drip out of it, but she spoke before we got in Eutaw.

"Well, wasn't it a pity and a shame that they had to come down there and break us up from seeing patients? We were saving them money to keep somebody from hiring somebody to drive them up to the clinic. They can come to Eutaw if they want to, and they can stay down there if they want to, because we were helping them. They weren't helping us."

I said, "Yes, ma'am." That's the only thing that come to me to say, "Yes, ma'am."

I never give it a thought when I get to talking. That's the way I was raised. A colored person is going to stay in his place. "Yes, ma'am." That's what I come up with. I was raised not to go too far, 'cause I might get something I didn't want. I held back because I knew night had to come.

My son told me, I could be broke. This boy of mine, what passed on, it would aggravate him so when I said, "Yes, sir and no, sir and yes, ma'am, and no, ma'am" to white folks.

I told my son, "You left home when you were seventeen years old. I still was here with Mama. You can't expect anything more of me."

But he couldn't stand it, 'cause he said, "In the army we slept together. We ate together. We waded trenches together, and why do I have to come back here and bow down, and say yes, sir, no, sir? I ain't going to do it."

But I say as little as possible, I put it that way. That's the only thing that come for me to say coming back to Eutaw. "Yes, ma'am." That was it. What I was thinking, I said that to myself. I keep that to myself, inside myself.

## Scratching out a Living

When I was working at the health department, I was still carrying my little farm, raising corn, peanuts, potatoes, stuff like that, and that's where I got my Social Security from. That's how come I'm sitting here today. Otherwise, I'd be out trying to find work. I expect I'd be out there begging.

Sometimes I got a good check, and sometimes I didn't. I just submitted hours that I put in. We had to turn our time in up here at the front desk when we get ready to come out. See, the health department wasn't cutting Social Security, and the midwife work was down. The only thing that helped me was I went to nursing white babies.

I went plenty places—Birmingham, Tuscaloosa, Mississippi, Georgia. I constantly just stayed in Birmingham, backwards and forth. After my name spread, there would always be somebody calling me, wanting me to come. I'd stay a week sometimes, sometimes two. Some babies be right cranky 'cause the mamas be nursing and the mamas ate up everything they see on the table. And whatever she eats, that baby is going to suck. Give them the colic, so help them.

There you are all night, one heel up in the air and the other one down. If you didn't have anybody washing dishes—just like you had a lady come in three times a week, the rest of them days, she would ask me to wash the dishes. That was extra time right there. But you had to take it and like it. That's the reason I said, it's good and bad.

Baby be three days old, and I take the baby in here, and it's in my room. Here's my bed, and here's the baby's bed over there. I'd stay two weeks. That's the only thing that helped me.

One time, I stayed three weeks for $150 a week. I usually stayed two. Sometimes you had to fix breakfast or supper and wash the baby's clothes, bed gown, and stuff like that. Keep your room clean.

One of the nurses was really nice to me and put an ad in the paper, and I started working then, sure enough. I thought I was doing something.

I remember the doctor getting me a job for a man and his wife living in a trailer. I rode down with him that evening after the clinic closed. He carried me in and introduced me to the people. He gave me his phone number before he left the office. If I have need for anything, call him, he said.

Everything was nice, but when I got there, the lady was already dressed. Her baby was four days old.

She told me, "Margaret, I'm going to the grocery store."

Before she left, she showed me where the milk and the bottles and water were. She showed me the room where me and the baby were going.

So she never showed up. Her husband, he came home from work. I was so upset by then, I didn't know what to say. I was with the baby, and as time went on, I kept a-looking for her.

He said, "Where did my wife go?"

I said, "I don't know."

He could have knocked my head off from me sitting up in there. All right, he went on to his mother and they stayed and stayed. He told me to fix myself some supper, but I yet ain't cooked nothing. I'm just sitting there.

Must I call the doctor? What must I do, 'cause you don't want to do the wrong thing. One mind said, "You call the doctor."

They stayed so long I was scared they might come back and catch me on the phone and wanting to know what I was doing. Sometimes, you have a vision. Your mind tells you, nothing will happen. I called him.

I said, "The mother left me with the baby. Said she was going to the grocery store about three o'clock, and she hasn't returned yet."

He said, "Where's the husband?"

I said, "He come by and asked me where his wife was, and I told him the same thing she told me."

The doctor said, "You reckon you can make it tonight?"

"I'll try. If he don't bother me, I sure ain't going to bother him."

He told me he'd see me in the morning about eight o'clock, and he was there a little bit before eight. He was smart. He didn't let on that I had told him or nothing.

I saw that black car coming in. He went on over to where the daddy was at the mother's house. The daddy was so slick he didn't come back that night. He didn't want to be in the trailer with just me and the baby.

I was looking right out the window at the doctor when he got out and knocked on the door. I could hear them talking. The woman was talking kind of slow and loud like. She said I had done my job all right. But that the woman was off to Florida, Indiana, or somewhere. She done parked that car at the bus station and left here. I ain't seen her from that day to this one. She quit him right there.

### Nursing the Elderly

During those late years I nursed babies, and I nursed old folks.

The boss man on the plantation, the white man I sassed, I nursed him. I nursed him a while when he was sick.

He told his wife, "Don't carry me nowhere. Margaret's going to wait on me."

Well, see, I reckon he felt like he treated me wrong, and he wanted to ask me to forgive him or something of the kind. You know, white folks is white, but his foot was just as blue as it could be.

He told me, "Margaret, I want you to wait on me 'cause you got patience, and you handle me just nice. Ain't nobody else going to do that."

I said, "All right, I appreciate you giving me that praise."

Anyhow, they put him in the hospital, but yet and still they had me to go to the hospital at night and sit with him. I stayed in the hospital with him till he got well, at night. He begged his wife, he said, "Margaret's going to wait on me."

I'd go every evening at five o'clock and come home at seven for twenty-four dollars a day. This was when things were starting to pick up. That was for working up at the hospital. See, he was crazy about me.

He just worried about me. When I left the hospital, his wife would tell me when I came back, "I'm so glad you came back, Margaret. Andy is about to worry me to death about you."

I said, "Ain't no use in worrying about me, I'm coming back on my time."

When I got there, he always wanted me to go straight in there. He'd say, "Do I hear Margaret's voice?"

But every time I looked at him I think 'bout how he would treat my husband and me, and not only me, but all the people on the plantation, all the way back up in there. I knew that, and every time I look at him, I'd think about it. But he just definitely wanted me to wait on him for some reason. He begged me. I guess he wanted me to forgive him or something of the kind.

## Freedom Now

Yes, we've come a long way, a mighty long way. People mostly have lights, and that makes a great difference, but I have been in many homes and they have to tote water, and the husband just working for a dollar a day, or a dollar twenty-five a day, or something like that. Folks just barely living.

We didn't know what credit cards were, nothing but lists—peck of meal, twenty-four-pound sack of flour, four pounds of lard, five pounds of sugar. And if you run out of anything, they let you get a half-gallon of syrup. You had to make do till the next time you come around. Had to last a month. Worked your ass all through the week. But you made it do, you had to. Sometimes you killed a chicken off the yard to help that meal out. People go to the blackberry patch, get some blackberries, and make a blackberry mummie [a fruit dumpling]. Now we have to buy that kind of stuff.

Back in time, people used to look at a dollar and think it was a ten-dollar bill. We picked cotton, plucked corn, we weren't making nothing, but then you can get something with nothing. Today you can't.

When Christmas come, you be lucky to get candy, an orange, or an apple. We took corn silk from corn and wrapped things. The boys used to make long sticks and walk up on them. Sometime, we had ribbon cane and sorghum. If you had an old cow, you had some milk. If you had a hog, you had some meat.

Now folks get where they can quit eating molasses and bread and go to meat and bread, they ought to thank God and

131

be humble, 'cause you don't know where you going to fall. When they get so they can put on a dress without a hole in it or a patch, get their hair fixed, they think they're Mr. Big.

But we used to couldn't go to town on Monday without the white man asking us what we doing there. Had to give an account.

I know the races halfway separated now, but before the marches, you couldn't go eat at the Eutaw Hotel. Even when people knew the civil rights had passed, and you could take a seat anywhere, but you still be asked out of that seat. Go to the back.

I'll tell you one thing they will still do right now. They'll take that white before they'll take you. I've seen that happen. The younger white race already looking back at the older race, 'cause they take white in there before they take you in. They take one thing paired with the other.

That's the reason I say, you might be there all morning, just like you have to make an appointment with a doctor to see him, and here come sits some white woman. She won't be sitting there five minutes before they call her in. There you sit now. Sometimes, it's just like that. Them old slave-time white folks, some of their younger race is here yet. All of them ain't dead.

It's not together like it should be. It's supposed to be if I'm white and you're colored or if you're white and I'm colored, if I cut you across your arm and you bleed, you can't bleed nothing but blood. It might be a different type, O or B or something of the kind, but it's still blood, ain't it? God made us all. See, if we are supposed to unite together, if we are supposed to be together in everything, we aren't supposed to go behind the curtain and talk about anything, if we don't have some colored person there. See what I mean? See, we know some things and some things, we never will know, way I see it.

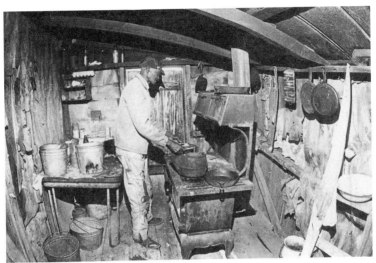

Clem Hicks, civil rights activist, Clinton, Greene County, c. 1968–69. Photo courtesy of Spiver Gordon.

They shouldn't put us behind in everything. We should have some of the blessings up here in front just like everybody else. We should have the say over some things. Yet and still, we've come a long ways. Let me say, I'm blessed from where I used to be. Sit anywhere on the plane. Sit anywhere on the bus. Some white folks killed themselves on account of it. We don't think where we've come from. People don't thank the Lord enough for how the Lord done blessed them. The colored folks don't have as much power as the white man, but we have more than we ever had.

See, I've been around too much. I've seen too much. I may look like a fool, but I'm not a fool, like way yonder of being one. See, I just watch the way you act. Anything and everything, I'm watching. Now you can just put that in your pocket, as my mama used to tell me, and sew it up.

| 6 |

# LAST DAYS

*By the 1980s, little remained* of the much maligned institution of black midwifery. After a century of grudging acceptance, Alabama, like other Deep South states, ceased issuing permits to "granny" midwives. A practice once considered natural became illegal.

The passage in 1976 of a new law governing the practice of nurse-midwives was the beginning of the end for traditional midwives. Black legislator Alvin Holmes cosponsored the bill, and he recalls little controversy surrounding its passage. While Act No. 499 specifically says, "Nothing in this section shall be construed as to prevent lay-midwives, holding valid health department permits, from engaging in the practice of lay-midwifery as heretofore provided until such time as said permit may be revoked by the County Board of Health," county health departments made renewal of lay-midwife permits extremely difficult. Physicians in some areas refused to sign midwife permits as required. Some county health departments rapidly "retired" midwives. For the first time, counties enforced health department guidelines requiring that no one over the age of sixty-five be allowed to practice midwifery. Even though a memo from Dr. Robert Goldenburg, state health department director of maternal and child health, indicated that midwives over sixty-five could continue to practice, with few exceptions, county health departments showed little flexibility in barring older

134

midwives from following their calling. After decades of practice, more than 150 Alabama midwives, all black, abruptly received letters and visits from physicians and nurses informing them that they could no longer work. Alabama placed severe strictures on a system that had included twenty-six hundred midwives in 1942. Each year all midwives had to renew their permits by April 10, but renewals became more and more difficult to get. No Alabama county health department issued a lay midwife permit after 1977. In one instance, a nurse casually dropped by the home of a midwife whose practice in Mobile County had begun in the 1920s, and told her that she was no longer a midwife. (The 1976 law also made it illegal for nurse-midwives to attend home births, and physicians who commonly did home deliveries in rural Alabama were growing older and facing new malpractice insurance coverage problems.)

Dr. Goldenburg responded to the growing concern about the implications of the nurse-midwife law for "granny" midwife practices on June 12, 1979, by issuing new guidelines: "No new granny midwives are to be certified after April 1, 1978." This meant that for the first time, women who were descendants of slave midwives could not continue their family tradition.

The end of lay midwifery met with little organized resistance. Lay midwives, typically older rural women, had no organization to fight for them. After decades of working under the supervision of local health departments, they found that they lacked the political means to develop advocates and allies. Midwife clubs sponsored by county health departments offered refresher courses, social events, and even religious services. They steered clear of political organizing and empowerment issues. Civil rights organizations and newly formed rural cooperatives, which addressed numerous grassroots economic issues, never rallied for midwives.

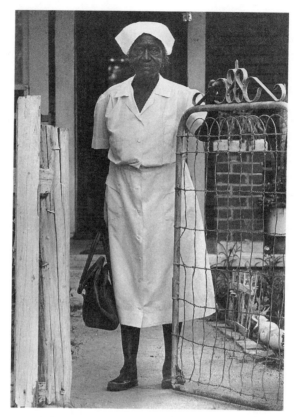

Aunt Shug, midwife, Coffee County, 1968. Photo by
Chester Higgins.

Many of these organizations still had a primarily male lead-
ership and continued to fight broad-based civil rights battles.
Newly formed lay-midwife organizations reached into the
Deep South only later on.

By the 1980s, women who had traditionally relied on, believed in, and preferred midwives were either beyond their
childbearing years or were going to hospitals to guarantee
insurance coverage. With the passage of Medicaid in 1965,

many traditional midwife clients turned to hospital-based medical care. (Medicaid did not reimburse lay midwives.) A new generation of childbearing women took their place. For them, midwives were associated with poverty, old-time ways, too few doctors, and segregation. Despite the growing tendency to respect traditional cultural expressions in the black community, there was no championing of traditional birthing practices as remnants of African or African American culture.

Dr. Sandral Hullett, a native of Birmingham, described the trend away from midwives:

> I understand that white women and black women used midwives for a certain period of time. Then as a person got more money, white or black, they used the doctor. As they got even more money they went to the hospital and that meant for many of the people right here that when our twenty-bed hospital opened, the majority of the people who delivered in the hospital were white. But as even they got more money, they would go to Tuscaloosa to the specialists and the obstetricians, because there are no obstetricians here. It's sort of been a status type of issue, an economical issue is the way I describe it. So the primary people in the group who didn't have any money were the black people in this area, and so they used what was available, and that was the lay midwife.

Some things changed with Medicaid, but poverty still persisted. More than a decade after the prohibition against lay midwives, 1990 census data indicated that the percentage of blacks living in poverty in Greene County is still higher than in any other county in the state. Stark white and black economic differences remain. The black poverty rate in Greene

County stands at 54.7 per 1,000; the white poverty rate, at 7.8 per 1,000.

## New-Age Births and Hospital Care

Ironically, just as Alabama was ending lay midwives' practices, the home birth movement was catching fire in feminist, consumer, and countercultural communities. Suddenly there was a middle-class market for midwives. One Alabama woman recalled how a white former resident of her small southern town flew her to a northeastern state to obtain her services as a midwife. Some private insurance companies even reimbursed lay midwives attending home births in Alabama. For the first time, traditional midwives, particularly in Alabama cities like Mobile and Huntsville, had growing numbers of private, third-party-insured, middle-class clients.

National (and mostly white) lay-midwifery organizations began to spring up. Nurse-midwifery organizations remained focused on their professional struggles to establish the scope of their practice and to define their position within the health care community. Many professional nurse-midwives came to respect lay midwives, as did some doctors. Beatrice Mongeau, a professional nurse-midwife in North Carolina, remembers learning from traditional midwives and recognizing the power of their community base. In a 1979 interview published by *Birth Gazette*, Alice Forman, a Eutaw nurse-midwife, argued, "I don't know as much about midwifery as Mrs. Smith does, because she has practiced for many years." Dr. Jesse Howard, a Selma doctor, similarly acknowledges midwifery skills, recalling how, in the 1960s, midwives taught him hand skills while he was completing a residency at the Tuskegee Institute. Dr. Howard hired traditional midwives to deliver babies in his office, but was forced to discontinue this practice because of pressure from county and state medical associations.

The opening of the Greene County rural health clinic in 1975 introduced comprehensive health care for the community, including preventive and prenatal care for families regardless of income. As federal guidelines raised the income limits for Medicaid eligibility, the poor had fewer problems in obtaining mainstream hospital care. When the county purchased its first ambulance in 1977, another barrier fell.

When these medical services first became available, Mrs. Smith was still an important resource for health care professionals. Dr. Hullett recalled, "We'd go and talk with Mrs. Smith. She worked a lot with us—the young women—and also she knew where a lot of different families lived and she helped us to get people in for care. So she was still an integral part of the health care system. Plus a lot of people in this community had delivered all their children at home. They didn't want to go to the hospital." Dr. Ruker Staggers recalls, "I signed Margaret's statement for a long time after anyone else. I guess she was one of the last in Alabama."

### Final Phase-Out

In 1981 the Alabama Department of Health sponsored its final midwife training conference at the Civic Center in downtown Montgomery. The marquees at the meeting site reading "Lay-Midwife Conference" lent a spurious glamor to an ill-paid, unappreciated, and misunderstood vocation. The midwives in attendance, dressed in their Sunday best or their immaculate white uniforms, were deeply concerned about their fate, but they had no forum in which to express their fears. Instead, they heard about how the new rules made their practices more difficult. Once again they found themselves subtly ridiculed for their lack of formal education, heard their skills questioned, and learned of strict enforcement of new regulations.

For traditional "granny" midwives the idea of maintaining their practices illegally or underground was not feasible. Defying the white medical power structure is riskier for them than it is for the new generation of midwives, who are willing to challenge the law. They are right to see their fate differently from that of the new generation of white midwives because of the century-long distrust demonstrated toward them by the medical system. Many of the older black midwives recognized that racial bias in the health care system, as in the criminal justice system, hindered opportunities for blacks. As some white midwives called on legal resources and strengthened ties with the political power structure, black midwives expected doors to be shut in their faces.

Direct-entry midwives are strong home-birth advocates who acquire their knowledge and skills independent of nurse-midwife educational programs. Several national groups support the home-birth movement and champion granting credentials to direct-entry midwives. (In a recent court case, a direct-entry midwife in Mobile was accused of homicide by the district attorney when the baby of a mother she was caring for was stillborn. She has won the support of the new statewide organization, Friends of Midwives, and her lawyers are considering seeking a U.S. Supreme Court ruling in this case).

For over a hundred years, the phasing out of traditional southern black midwives was said to be the key to lowering high infant mortality rates. Beatrice Mongeau, a white nurse-midwife practicing in Maryland in the 1950s, recalled taking part in that state's early efforts to phase out midwives. She found, however, that her experiences with the midwives were positive:

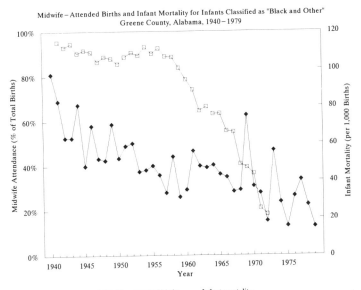

Midwife – Attended Births and Infant Mortality for Infants Classified as "Black and Other"
Greene County, Alabama, 1940 – 1979

NOTE: Midwife attendance data are not available for 1940 and 1973 – 1979
SOURCE: Alabama Department of Public Health

My job was to eliminate the granny midwife. If they weren't so powerful in their communities, I would have overcome them. Depression was a factor, and the war was a factor. I remember kids coming from New York just to have the midwife because they couldn't afford to have their babies any other way. I ended up having the deepest respect for them. We learned from each other. I realized we needed the midwives to work with us. Otherwise the women in the community would not listen to us. We even had prenatal clinics at the midwives' homes. It was the only way to get some of the mothers to come for prenatal care.

In Greene County, infant mortality was admittedly high, but it did not consistently correlate with percentages of

141

midwife-attended births. Alice Forman, who worked alongside Mrs. Smith in the public health clinic, noted that the problem of high infant mortality rates persisted even when midwives did few births. While midwife-attended births declined steadily, as figures from 1941 to 1972 show, sporadic rises in infant mortality have occurred. During one period infant mortality rates declined faster than midwife attendance. Fluctuations in infant mortality are certainly due to multiple factors, of which lay-midwife attendance may or may not be one.

According to a recent analysis of national infant mortality published in the *American Journal of Public Health*, significant racial disparities in maternal and infant outcomes across educational and income differences have widened in recent years. It is now recognized that declines in infant mortality rates since the 1950s are related to drops in mortality from pneumonia and influenza, respiratory distress syndrome, prematurity and low birthweight, congenital anomalies, and accidents. Although infant mortality has dropped dramatically in Alabama, the state still lacks accessible prenatal care in several counties. This may explain why, according to the *1990 Alabama Vital Events*, the state's infant mortality rate is among the highest in the nation. That year, Pickens County, neighbor to Greene County, had the state's highest infant mortality rate: 35.7 per 1,000 live births for the total population and 48.8 per 1,000 live births for blacks.

Most maternal and child health experts agree that addressing the problem of poor maternal and infant outcomes requires a multifaceted approach that includes such social remedies as education, jobs, and housing as well as nutritional support and treatment of alcohol, smoking, and drug problems. A North Carolina study comparing birth outcomes where lay midwives working with health departments were in attendance to outcomes where physicians were present found that black "granny" midwives compared favorably to doctors. A comprehensive health care team addressed the medical concerns of women in need of specialized care, and the health care system provided appropriate emergency support for all women.

Today, Alabama women remain without the right to choose a midwife for a home birth. Four of the five states showing a decrease in midwifery births between 1975 and 1988 were in the South; the decline was mostly among black mothers. In 1995 midwives attended 4.9 percent of all births in the United States, but most of these midwives were hospital-based nurse-midwives. One nurse-midwife practicing in Alabama, recently reflected, "If you have the right to die at home, one would think you have the right to be born at home."

The School of Nursing at the University of Alabama in Birmingham established the state's first and only nurse-midwife educational program in 1990. Its doors closed six years later when monumental barriers for obtaining clinical experience and licensure turned the nurse-midwife program into a new-age dinosaur. As Marilyn Musacchio, the university's nurse-midwife educational director, explained, "Students faced enormous difficulties finding adequate clinical experience in Birmingham and across the state." Dr. Musacchio added that the few students who did graduate were discouraged from practicing in Alabama. With one of the nation's most stringent nurse-midwife licensing regulations, Alabama requires a nurse-midwife to find a physician who regularly delivers babies to sponsor her for licensure. If a nurse-midwife changes practice sites within her community or moves to another part of the state, she must find a new sponsor. A doctor can sponsor only one nurse-midwife at a time, and today, with thirty-three counties in Alabama having no hospitals with maternity wards, nurse-midwives have difficulty finding practicing maternity physicians. The Alabama nurse-practice act is now under review, and it remains unclear if new regulations will grant nurse-midwives any more freedom. Regardless of the outcome of the review, the state's only educational program did not survive, graduating its last nurse-midwife class in June 1996.

Similarly, exactly two decades earlier, time and circumstances worked against Mrs. Smith and other black midwives. The Alabama Medical Society, the state health department, and the legislature made no attempt to distinguish more experienced midwives from the women who only occasionally attended births. Studies compared infant mortality rates only by place of birth—in hospital or out of hospital—ignoring the many factors that influence birth outcomes. The statistics do not even differentiate between accidental emergency deliveries and planned home births. In the last years of lay midwifery, the tests and other measurements of midwifery skill continued to reflect white cultural bias and failed to explore alternative ways of substantiating midwifery knowledge. Midwives never had a hand in designing tools for self-measurement of skills, for example. The people who designed and administered tests for midwives were not interested in alternative ways of recognizing midwifery skills. The World Health Organization, in contrast, has developed tools for measuring the proficiency of diverse types of birth attendants. These measurements are seldom used in the United States, which tends to reject caregivers who cannot demonstrate their skills on standard examinations.

In Alabama midwives were caught in a double bind when they failed to measure up in their use of some basic instruments. Once again issues of control and of racial bias became a major roadblock for midwives. In the last years of their practice they were criticized for failing to use blood pressure cuffs—but the county health departments refused to train them in their use, claiming that only nurses should use them.

Fortunately, southern black communities never depended on institutional medicine to define their midwifery icons. In fact, one Alabama town, Childersburg, named its urban renewal project in honor of Mrs. Sadie Lee, who attended nearly two thousand births in Talladega County. The *Childersburg Star* said that Mrs. Lee "did more for her people than any other person who ever lived in this area." Although increasingly vulnerable over the decades, midwives survived because their care was needed and wanted. The lives of midwives like Mrs. Smith are pictures of how strong spirits stand tall in the face of the scorn that strikes like a whip on a slave's back. Medical biases, shallow analysis, and outright racial affronts do not change her self-perception. Mrs. Smith's spirit comes from herself and from her neighbors, and she fearlessly tells her story in this book. As one of the "old heads," she speaks like a soothsayer in a modern-day wilderness. Her warnings about the inappropriateness of today's medically managed high-tech births are the knobkerry stick with which she once again summons folks to "listen good."

ALL THEY WANTED WAS the midwives off. Training was the last thing they wanted. They wrote me at the health department that I couldn't be no more midwife. I had to bring my bag and my equipment in, not only me, but all of them that was delivering.

But I think Dr. Staggers helped me as long as he could. I have to give him credit for that. He would let people come through with their girls fixing to have a baby. Some of them have their babies out there in the front yard, in the car. Then I'd have to get on the phone to call him. He'd tell me to fix them up, carry them on home, and come on by the office.

This girl who had the baby in the front yard told me, "I started to Tuscaloosa. But my daughter was having pains so fast, I decided to turn around and come back to you."

I said, "Who's the doctor?"

She told me, "Dr. Staggers."

I said, "I have to call him before I can do anything for you, or you talk to him."

I called, and that baby come. That was called underground. I reckon I did that for so long, and then I quit because people began to talk.

"You know Margaret? She delivered that gal's baby over there."

But every once in a while, I'd come across a young girl that's on Medicaid. She wanted to stay at home because she's afraid to go to the hospital. I'll tell you this, it was the people who are not on Medicaid that are usually the ones that looked for me, because they'd have to have the hundred dollars before they'd get admitted to the hospital. Of course, if you don't have it, you are going to have to sit out there in your chair in the waiting room, and you'll have to go back and find somebody else. You'll have to find a midwife.

I've carried them to the doctor and had to carry them back home even when the doctor said they couldn't have the baby at home. We had them in the middle of the road.

Dr. Staggers, he kept me. They kept pushing him to get rid of me, but after a while, Dr. Staggers told me to come by during the week, if I had the time. He wanted to do some special talk to me. He said, "Margaret, I hate to tell you what I'm going to tell you, but I've gone as far as I can go holding you in Greene County. I am going to have to let you go. You're a

146

good midwife. I'm sorry. I'd put you up beside anybody in delivering a baby."

Dr. Staggers, he's so kind.

I said, "I was expecting it to come, because they cut off all the midwives but me."

He just had to come up and tell me. Tears were in his eyes. He hated it so bad to see me go. I had to go. We didn't have no more midwives. That was the end of the midwives.

Everybody goes to the hospital now. Some of them feel pretty good about it, and some don't. But if you go to the hospital, you're going to pay some money.

The doctors have made them so much money. They take two thousand, three thousand for delivering one baby. That's a lot of money, and you're doing all the work.

The way I look at it, you just as soon stay home and have your baby, if possible, if you are in good health and don't have problems. Some women just can't because something just flares up wrong.

I think it's just better to stay home than to go to the hospital. Go to the hospital, have your baby, get up and go home the next day? I'd have the baby at home and let that do.

You can have your way more at home. You have your own freedom at home. You won't have to lay down until your time come. You can get up and do things. The baby won't have to be drugged before birth from giving you those shots to knock you out.

I tell you one thing: These doctors are tired of delivering so many colored babies, not white but colored. They say, we are tired of the colored babies 'cause the mothers are from fifteen, even twelve years old. That's the reason you won't see a doctor in the delivery room that much.

The nurse is the one who delivers the baby. They catch the baby. The doctors don't even be in there. Sometimes you have the baby by yourself. You holler and buck and rear until the baby comes. Some of the ladies, when they first started going to the hospital, they strapped you down and wouldn't allow you anything to eat. Right now, ladies going to the hospital say the doctor may look at you, feel your stomach, then out the door he goes.

But these mothers, they still rather be in the hospital where they can whoop and holler, thinking the doctor is going to give them something to ease them pains, but the doctors won't be there. The nurse be back there, and they come in there every occasion. You need somebody back there with you. Now a midwife, she's got to be right there, sitting right aside the bed or sitting over you, holding you, rocking you, rubbing you.

### Distant Justice

It's a hard struggle. It doesn't look like Alabama is going to get the midwives back. We had a nurse-midwife once who had been working in Jackson, Mississippi. The head of the health department got her to come to Greene County.

I said, all right, that be good, but she never got to really work. Most of the doctors wouldn't let her work under them. The head doctors were saying, you-all midwives got to go. She came and never did get a chance to deliver ne'er a baby by herself. She hated that 'cause she couldn't do what she was trained to do.

Now I believe the young race, the young doctors, would go for the white midwives more so than they would the colored because they don't want the colored people to have nothing nohow but scrubbing floors and washing windows. I think the white midwives would have a better chance.

If they say that we're going to let midwives come back to Alabama, supposed to be getting our licenses, our equipment today, we'll be the last to know it. The white midwives will be there, and got what they wanted when we find out about it. Well, where does that put you? Behind, doesn't it? You're going to be behind on and on.

If they do bring the midwives back, some of us will be done got so rusty, we won't know what we did when they cut us off. All right, say, I did go to school over in Selma to become a nurse-midwife. I have to be gone a year for nursing training. All right, what's going to come of my house? My things are here. I got to have somebody here while I'm over there.

All right, I get graduated. I get my diploma and everything to go with it. Here I come back, a nurse-midwife. I've lost a whole year now.

All right, somebody comes strutting along and says, "I'm going to the hospital like I've been going."

Here I come out of school, and I'm waiting on you thinking that you might tell me that now you'd love to have me.

But she'd still say, "I don't want that woman nohow. I'm going to the hospital like I've been going to have my baby unless they turn me down there. That will be the only way that I'll come back and have anything to do with you."

I've saved more babies, but they're losing a whole lot of babies now. There is more red tape to it now than it was when we were working. You could count on midwives. They took care of everybody, no matter what.

That's the reason why I wondered why they cut the midwives off. Just turned us a-loose, half paid, nothing. Just turned us a-loose, and said, "This is your last day."

I think it's awful the way they did us. If they come back, midwives will have to do this type of nursing work in the hospital because they don't want you no way to do midwife work nohow, too much responsibility on them. See, it's all up to the doctors.

Back when I was still working, the younger ones said, no, they didn't want to be no midwife. They just didn't want this midwife work. How much they pay?

See, they'd been 'round people having babies and saw how long the midwife had to sit there, stay there. Didn't have nothing to eat. If you ate something that made you sick, then that was you.

I would go back to midwife, if those drugs just weren't so heavy. Midwife pays pretty good now from what it used to be. It wasn't nothing then. Now it's pretty good money. But the mothers take so much drugs, drug city, Tuscaloosa, that's what I'm scared of, and AIDS.

One girl down here, they said they picked up the vacuum cleaner and the rats fell out. The roaches had a picnic. Well, that ain't no way. I just couldn't live, wouldn't live nowhere where I couldn't live clean and decent.

And then every year one or two people come out the North, every year to come home to die of AIDS.

But I tell you what, I wouldn't have it now if they were paying five hundred dollars a baby, 'cause you see there's so much of AIDS, and folks ain't going to tell you the truth, and before you know anything you got AIDS, fooling with you. That's right. You'll never know. I wouldn't go through it no more for my weight in gold.

I knew the responsibility was left in my hand whenever I hit the house, and I had to try to do my part. I felt like if I didn't, well, that was it. That's the way I felt. And then I guess the Lord had something to do with it. I felt like that. If you can help somebody, help them. Don't go there and just sit down and cross your legs and get you a book and reading it, uh-uh. You had to do what you could. The way I felt about it, that was the making up of the job or any job you go on. You have to try to do it right, and I've seen so many tricks pulled that it ain't even funny, working.

If you had the baby all right, no complaint, no hurting nowhere or fainting or what have you, everything going well, I know I'd soon be ready to go home. That's what made me happy. I'd just tell her to be good and try to take care of herself until I get back.

Plenty times, I come out the field and didn't get my supper done before somebody came looking for me, after me. I'd be so tired till I couldn't hardly stand up to take a bath. Be done worked hard all day and going to sit up all night long.

It would be bad if I got into something, nowhere I can go. I'd have to hurry up and get out of Greene County and parts of other cities. Some place like Tuscaloosa, a lot of people in Tuscaloosa know me—Demopolis, Greensboro, Montgomery, all around. I delivered babies all over Greene County till you get to the Sumter County line, Mantua, Union, Gena, up to Ralph. I went that far. I didn't have any business up there, but I went. People were just wild about me. I thought I was doing a big thing. Midwifing used to be our job. That and going to field.

## Moving On

Now most of the people are gone. They moved away when the civil rights movement started. The colored people just scattered like birds.

The head doctors who accepted midwives when I was growing up, they're dead and gone. The first ten years I worked, they thought the midwife was very important 'cause they didn't have no other choice. But since all this health department thing come along—nurse going out to see you, you going into the clinic, and they telling you that you can't have a midwife—you got to have a doctor. Well, they got that through their heads, and that's what they did. I didn't want to be a midwife in the first place, but I appreciated the work. I think it would be good if midwives could have kept on practicing, 'cause one day all this is going to be banished away, and you're going to have to go back to the midwife.

If they do like they did when I came through, I'm telling you, it's going to be tough. If it's as tough as it was when I was on, I don't want nothing at it, and I expect it's going to be worse. It's going on back there now. If they do like when I was going through, it's going to be tough.

I'll be ninety the twelfth of September [1996], if I live to see. I don't know when my time will come. You just got to keep on looking, looking to the hills.

When John asked the Master when was he going to die, God told John to shut the book.

That means you ain't supposed to know. Be a terrible thing to know. But when you're dead and gone, you're dead and gone.

The way I feel about it, like the person who is here that is my age, and with the mind I got, I have done good deeds back. I could have done like Dennis. I could have left home when I got grown, but my heart just wouldn't go that way.

I kept my uncle till he died. I helped see after my husbands' folks till they died. So I think the Lord is blessing me for it. Like I before told you, there ain't but three [two] of my playmates left that I knew when I was coming up, going to school. That's me, Annie Lee James, and Florence Dunlap Hicks. That's all that's left. Even now some of their children and things is dead and gone. Florence had three, but her girl's

152

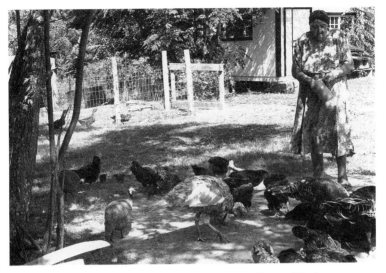

Mrs. Smith feeding poultry, 1995. Photo by Sharon Blackmon.

dead, and her son is dead, and I don't know how many Anna Lee got living. Just a blessing to be here, and I thank the Lord for it, 'cause I declare, Lord, there's been so many folks gone on since I've been here. Me, Florence, and Annie Lee is a big setup of people, a big family. Garvin Cockrell is dead. Mamie Cockrell is dead. Kevin dead. Miss Rose dead, and William dead. All the old folks just about played out from here.

But I can think way back, and that's a blessing. I can tell people what I know, I know it, I ain't forgot it, and I'm not ashamed to tell it either, and that's a blessing. I could be sitting in this chair and couldn't get out, or in a rolling chair.

I'm not doing nothing now but keeping house and trying to see to my cows. I don't have a hog, but I'm going to try to buy me one. Sometimes I get bored 'cause I don't like to be in the way of other people, going to their house and sitting down. So I just sit here and turn the TV on. If I get me some glasses,

I'm going on to piecing quilt. But I don't have too long to sit down, though. I have my ironing to do, and my washing to do, and changing beds. I have all that to do. I could do anything I've ever done, if it weren't for my leg. I just can't get along like I used to.

Most Sundays I don't go to church. These days the people done got so full of pot. I tell you, about the biggest thing now is money. The deacon, he's stealing, and the preacher is getting his part, too. They don't mind asking us for twenty-five, thirty, forty, fifty, men's a hundred, some women a hundred. I said, my Lord, you got to wait till I get a hundred!

Now I can have Christmas any day I get ready. Cook chicken. Cook ham. Get me some fruit. Make one or two cakes. I can have me some Christmas. The young race ain't going to do what we done. The children just didn't grow up that way. There's going to be a lot of killing, I reckon, 'cause they ain't going to do what we done. See, greens and cornbread don't do me no harm. But just like the colored people they won't work from eighteen, nineteen years old. How you going to eat? Where you going to sleep? You got to have a way made somehow or another. If you break in these white folks' places, and they catch you, then they going to kill you. And there ain't no jobs to amount to shit. Ain't going to be no jobs to amount to nothing. Ain't going to be like it is now. It's coming on down.

It's been forty years since the Republicans been in the House. They're going to be raising sand. Back in time, I had to make it some way for my children. So I had to get. I had to walk from here to Eutaw. That's the reason my legs ain't no 'count now. I leave here around five o'clock in the morning. I'd be there way before seven. It didn't take me long to walk it, but if I had known I was damaging myself in this day in time, I don't know. I reckon I'd of toughed it on out. But see, like I told you, there weren't no cars or nothing, just them mules, wagons, horses and buggies.

Very seldom you see a colored person with a wagon and horse. Prisoners would be working on the road with shackles on their feet. Ice be shooting up out the ground like my arm. Shackles on their legs like they going to do now. They got them in some places already, got shackles on them.

I just think the younger race having babies now don't be what the elder people, the old heads, used to be. Now take motherwit and book learning, two different things. I got more motherwit and not as much of an education 'cause we had to go to field.

I was raised to learn a little of everything I could learn possible, because you don't know when it's going to come around that you may have to do some of these things. This way, it won't go so hard with you, when you have to do it.

I say the children got so much of freedom now, they don't try to learn these different things. They don't try to learn how to cook. They don't try to learn how to wash. They don't try to learn how to iron. It would be a blessing for the young race to learn these old things. My grandmother, who was brought to this country and sold, taught me everything I know. She knew these things because she come from Africa, and she was a big old girl, the way she talked, when they brought her to this country. I guess aplenty of things she had already seen the people do. I think that's how she knew these things.

I had a paper that I wouldn't take a million dollars for, if I still had it. It got burned up when my house caught on fire. It stated who bought Mama and what year she was brought to this country and sold. I had it in the Bible, family Bible, but it all got burned up. The old log house caught on fire right down from here. These old tricks and different things that's in me, it'll be in me till death. These things are not too hard to learn.

155

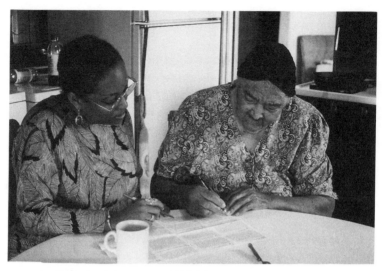

Authors signing contract, 1995. Photo by Charles Robertson.

But the young race ain't trying to learn. They know it all. Nothing that you can't learn. You can learn these things. You don't ever know what you got to come to. Oh, I have been through it, been through the wringer, but I did what the Lord wanted me to do 'cause the Lord loves his people, especially children. I rode many a night in wagons. Then I have to wade water to my knees getting to the people's homes. Come a big rain, like it would start raining about four o'clock and rain on till eight or nine, and I had to get up and leave home and go out. I had to wade water where a wagon or buggy couldn't get across.

I'm worth millions of dollars for what I've done done. I thought I was doing a big thing. I was proud of it. The lives that I've saved, going to deliver all these babies, till I got something to be thankful for. The children have grown so. Some of them have to bend their heads down to hardly get in that door. They have grown just that way. I am thankful, yeah.

# EPILOGUE

*Mrs. Smith continues* to live at home in Eutaw, Alabama, with her two sons, Houston and Herman. Swelling in her legs and feet requires her to make frequent trips to the doctor. Family, neighbors, and friends, white and black, keep a caring and watchful eye on Mrs. Smith. Her phone rings often, and she has regular visitors who bring freshly killed chickens, vegetables from the garden, and good conversation. One of Mrs. Smith's favorite pastimes remains a good discussion about the way things used to be. She believes folks should look back before looking ahead. Mrs. Smith is proud that her old-time ways include mastering such arts of the home as making a good pound cake and fixing a comfortable bed for guests. Around sundown Mrs. Smith can be found yodeling for her cows to come eat their feed. The short drive from her house to town is a major outing for Mrs. Smith. On every trip to the A & P with Mrs. Smith I get spontaneous testimonials to her, because so many people have so much that's positive to say. As for now, Mrs. Smith looks forward to receiving lots of mail from folks who read this book. Her address is Route 3, Box 220, Eutaw, Alabama 35462.

During my last phone conversation with Mrs. Smith on this book, I realized there are still unwritten volumes in her. One chapter might be on the power of the mind. Recently, even though no one had told her about it, she sensed trouble in a friend's life, and her mental energies remained focused on him. Mrs. Smith believes, "Whatever my mind lies on, it's there. I'm staying on it." She told me she is using her mind to reach him with the message, "It's better to eat shit with the chickens than to just sit there and let somebody do you wrong." With her longest road behind her, Mrs. Smith accepts not knowing when or where the Lord will call her home. Victory is believing her mind/spirit delights in defying earthly space and time.

I remain particularly interested in the documentation of black midwifery and its resistance to assimilating the ways of mainstream medicine. Anyone interested in contributing to efforts to preserve black Alabama birthing lore and arti-facts—record books, birthing tools, photographs, and other items having to do with midwifery—should write Linda Janet Holmes c/o West Alabama Health Services, P.O. Box 711, Eutaw, Alabama 35462.

For more information on midwives, home birth, and birth centers, contact the following organizations:


Alabama Friends of Midwives
P.O. Box 892
Daphne, Alabama, 36526


The American College of Nurse-Midwives
818 Connecticut Ave. NW, Suite 900
Washington, D.C. 20006
(202) 728-9860

Births, Books, and Beyond
2472 Douglass Avenue
New York, New York 10027
(212) 694-1929


Midwives Association of North America (MANA)
P.O. Box 175
Newton, Kansas 67114
(316) 283-4543

# BIBLIOGRAPHY

Alabama Department of Public Health. *Midwife Manual.* Montgomery, 1936.

———. Center for Health Statistics. *1990 Alabama Vital Events.* Rev. ed. Montgomery, 1992.

Alabama Industrial Development Board. *Industrial Survey of Greene County.* Birmingham, 1930.

"Alabama's Midwifery Problem." *Journal of the Medical Association of the State of Alabama* 3 (1933): 148–49.

Alley, Kristie. "Ruck Staggers: Country Doctor." *Tuscaloosa News,* 11 October 1992, p. 1.

Andriot, John L. *Population Abstract of the United States.* McLean, Virginia: Andriot Associates, 1983.

Borst, Charlotte G. *Catching Babies: The Professionalization of Childbirth, 1870–1920.* Cambridge: Harvard University Press, 1996.

Boston Women's Health Collective. *The New Our Bodies Ourselves.* New York: Simon and Schuster, 1984.

Boston Women's Health Book Collective, National Black Women's Health Network, and the Women's Institute for Childbearing Policy. "Excerpt from Childbearing Policy within a National Health Program: An Evolving Consensus for New Directions." In *Women's Health: Readings on Social, Economic, and Political Issues,* 2d ed., edited by Nancy Worcester and Marianne H. Whatley. Dubuque, Iowa: Kendall/Hunt, 1994.

Bouleware, Thomas M. "Transactions of the Association: Maternal and Child Health." *Journal of the Medical Association of the State of Alabama* 18 (1949): 311–12.

Bovard, Wendy, and Gladys Milton. *Why Not Me? The Story of Gladys Milton, Midwife.* Summertown, Tennessee: Book Publishing Company, 1993.

Brown, S. S. Kirksey, Foster M., Correspondence, 11 February 1865. W. Stanley Hoole Special Collections Library. University of Alabama Libraries.

Burnett, Claude A., III, James A. Jones, Judith Rooks, Chong Hwa Chen, Carl W. Tyler Jr., and Arden C. Miller. "Home Delivery and Neonatal Mortality in North Carolina." *Journal of the American Medical Association* 244 (1980): 2741–45.

Campbell, Marie. *Folks Do Get Born.* New York: Rinehart and Company, 1946.

Carmer, Carl. *Stars Fell on Alabama.* Rahway, New Jersey: Quinn and Boden, 1934.

Clark, Joanna. "Motherhood." In *The Black Woman: An Anthology,* edited by Toni Cade Bambara. New York: Doubleday, 1970.

Committee on Maternal and Infant Welfare. "Transactions of the 1935 Session—Part 1." *Journal of the Medical Association of the State of Alabama* 5 (1935): 25–26.

———. "Transactions of the 1937 Session—Part 1." *Journal of the Medical Association of the State of Alabama* 7 (1937): 30–31.

Coombs, David W., M. H. Alsikafi, C. Hobson Bryan, and Irving L. Webber. "Black Political Control in Greene County, Alabama." *Rural Sociology* 42 (1977): 398–406.

Crellin, John K., and Jane Philpott. *Herbal Medicine Past and Present.* Vol. 1, *Trying to Give Ease.* Durham, N.C.: Duke University Press, 1990.

Cunningham, William A. "Bureau of Maternal and Child Health: Maternity Care." *Journal of the Medical Association of the State of Alabama* 14 (1944): 51–52.

Davis, Charles T., ed. *Strange Ways and Sweet Dreams: Afro-American Folklore from the Hampton Institute.* Boston: G. K. Hall, 1983.

Davis, Lorna. "The Use of Castor Oil to Stimulate Labor in Patients with Premature Rupture of Membranes." *Journal of Nurse-Midwifery* 29 (1984): 366–70.

Davis, Sheila, and Cora A. Ingram. "Empowered Caretakers: A Historical Perspective on the Roles of Granny Midwives in Rural Alabama." In *Wings of Gauze: Women of Color and the Experience of Health and Illness,* edited by Barbara Bair and Susan Cayleff, 191–201. Detroit: Wayne State University Press, 1993.

"A Death in the Family: Alabama's Infant Mortality Crisis." *Alabama Journal,* September 14–18, 1987.

Declercq, Eugene R. "The Transformation of American Midwifery: 1975 to 1988." *American Journal of Public Health* 82 (1992): 680–84.

Dibble, Eugene H., Louis A. Raab, and Ruth B. Ballard. "Original Communications: John A. Andrew Memorial Hospital." *Journal of the National Medical Association* 53 (1961): 103–18.

Dodson, R. B. "Some Obstetrical Experiences of a Country Doctor." *Transactions of the Medical Association of the State of Alabama* (1927): 169–73.

Fisher, Brad. "Greene County Gets an Ambulance." *Tuscaloosa News,* 1 June 1977, p. 28.

Fitzgerald, Michael W., "To Give Our Votes to the Party: Black Political Agitation and Agricultural Change in Alabama, 1865–1870." *Journal of American History* 76 (1989): 489–94.

Foster, Steven, and James A. Duke. *A Field Guide to Medicinal Plants.* Boston: Houghton Mifflin, 1990.

Frankel, Barbara. *Childbirth in the Ghetto: Folk Beliefs of Negro Women in a North Philadelphia Hospital Ward.* San Francisco: R & E Research Associates, 1977.

Fraser, Gertrude J. "Modern Bodies, Modern Minds: Midwifery and Reproductive Change in an African American Community." In *Conceiving the New World Order: The Global Politics of Reproduction*, edited by Faye D. Ginsberg and Rayna Rapp, 42–57. Berkeley: University of California Press, 1995.

Garrison, J. E. "Delivering Babies at Home." *Journal of the Medical Association of the State of Alabama* 12 (1943): 228–31.

Gaskin, Ina May. *Spiritual Midwifery*. 3d ed. Summertown, Tennessee: Book Publishing Company, 1990.

——. "Why Was This Woman's Job Taken Away?" *Birth Gazette* 8 (1992): 28–30.

Gentry, Diane Koos. *Enduring Women*. College Station: Texas A & M University Press, 1988.

Goldenberg, Robert, Christiane Hale, John Houde, Joan Humphrey, John Wayne, and Beverly Boyd. "Neonatal Deaths in Alabama." *American Journal of Obstetrics and Gynecology* 147 (1983): 687–93.

Gray, Fred. *Bus Ride to Justice: Changing the System by the System*. Montgomery, Alabama: Black Belt Press, 1995.

Greene, Melissa. "All the Hours of the Night: The Recollections of a Country Midwife." *Country Journal* (November 1987): 58–66.

Grime, William Ed. *Ethno-Botany of the Black Americans*. Algonac, Michigan: Reference Publications, 1979.

Hampton, Henry, Steve Frayer, and Sarah Flynn, compilers. *Voices of Freedom: An Oral History of the Civil Rights Movement from the 1950s to the 1980s*. New York: Bantam, 1990.

Harlan, Louis R., ed. *Booker T. Washington Papers*. Vol. 3, *1889–95*. Urbana: University of Illinois Press, 1974.

Harris, Kate. "Greene County Victory More Historic than Moon Walk, Abernathy." *Birmingham Post Herald*, 31 July 1969, p. 6.

Hennessey, Melinda Meek. "Political Terrorism in the Black Belt: The Eutaw Riot." *Alabama Review* 33 (1980): 35–48.

Holmes, Linda Janet. "African American Midwives in the South." In *The American Way of Birth*, edited by Pamela S. Eakins, 273–91. Philadelphia: Temple University Press, 1986.

———. "Alabama Granny Midwives." *Journal of the Medical Society of New Jersey* 81 (1984): 389–91.

———. "Thank You Jesus to Myself: The Life of a Traditional Black Midwife." In *The Black Woman's Health Book*, edited by Evelyn C. White, 98–106. Seattle: Seal Press, 1990.

Houde, John, Joan L. Humphrey, Beverly W. Boyd, and Robert L. Goldenberg. "Out of Hospital Deliveries in Alabama 1940–1980." *Journal of the Medical Association of the State of Alabama* (April 1982): 20–23.

Howe, Marvin. "Antebellum Charm in Alabama." *New York Times*, 21 March 1993, Travel section.

Hullett, Sandral. "Where a Ride to the Doctor Costs $20." *Aging* no. 359 (1989): 14–16.

Ityavyar, Dennis A. "A Traditional Midwife Practice, Sokoto State, Nigeria." *Social Science Medicine* 18 (1984): 497–501.

Iweze, Felicia Apenasami. "Taboos of Childbearing and Childrearing in Bendel State of Nigeria." *Journal of Nurse-Midwifery* 28 (1983): 31–33.

Jackson, Lynne. "The Production of George Stoney's Film *All My Babies: A Midwife's Own Story* (1952)." *Film History* 1 (1987): 367–92.

Jacobson, Paul H. "Hospital Care and the Vanishing Midwife," *Milbank Memorial Fund Quarterly* 34 (1956): 253–61.

Jacoby, Karl. "From Plantation to Hacienda: The Mexican Colonization Movement in Alabama." *Alabama Heritage* 35 (1995): 34–43.

Johnson, Charles S. *Statistical Atlas of Southern Counties Listing and Analysis of Socio-Economic Indices of 1104 Southern Counties.* Chapel Hill: University of North Carolina Press, 1941.

Johnson, Halle T. "The La Fayette Dispensary." *Report of Proceedings of the Nineteenth Annual Meeting of the Alumnae*

*Association of the Women's Medical College of Pennsylvania.*
9–10 May 1894.

Jones, Jacqueline. *Labor of Love, Labor of Sorrow: Black Women, Work, and the Family from Slavery to the Present.* New York: Vintage Books, 1985.

Jones, James H. *Bad Blood: The Tuskegee Syphilis Experiment.* New York: Free Press, 1981; new edition, revised and expanded, 1993.

Jones, Paul, M.D. "Problems in Country Practice." *Transactions of the Medical Association of the State of Alabama* (1927): 166–68.

Jordan, Brigitte. *Birth in Four Cultures,* 3d ed. Montreal: Eden Press, 1983.

Jordan, Ed. "State's Infant Mortality A Continuing Concern." *The* (Greene County) *Democrat,* 26 May 1993, p. 1.

Kenney, John A., M.D. *The Negro in Medicine.* Tuskegee University Archives, 1912.

Kirschenfeld, J. J. *No Greater Privilege.* Montgomery, Alabama: Black Belt Press, 1992.

Kline, Anna. "'With Them I Wouldn't Be Lookin' No Shame': Models of Medical Decision-Making among Rural Alabama Black Women." Ph.D. diss., Rutgers University, 1984.

Knutson, Richard A., Lloyd Merbitz, Maurice Creekmore, and Gene H. Snipes. "Use of Sugar and Povidone-Iodine to Enhance Wound Healing: Five Years' Experience." *Southern Medical Journal* 74 (1981): 1329–35.

Laderman, Carol. *Wives and Midwives: Childbirth and Nutrition in Rural Malaysia.* Berkeley: University of California Press, 1987.

Levine, Lawrence. *Black Culture and Black Consciousness.* Oxford: Oxford University Press, 1977.

"Life in Greene County Little Changed in 100 Years." *Birmingham Post Herald,* 22 February 1977, p. A9.

Litoff, Judy Barrett. *American Midwives, 1860 to the Present.* Westport, Connecticut: Greenwood Press, 1978.

Litwak, Leon F. *Been in the Storm So Long: The Aftermath of Slavery.* New York: Alfred A. Knopf, 1979.

Logan, Onnie Lee, as told to Katherine Clark. *Motherwit: An Alabama Midwife's Story.* New York: E. P. Dutton, 1989.

McWhorter, Diane. "Celebrity Time down South." *The Nation,* 1 February 1986, pp. 109–12.

Magin, Janis L. "Lay Midwives Made to Labor in Shadows." *Montgomery Advertiser,* 6 May 1994, p. 1.

Marriner, Jessie L. "Midwifery in Alabama." Unpublished manuscript in the Rockefeller Foundation Library (1925?).

Maternity Center Association. *Twenty Years of Nurse-Midwifery, 1933–1953.* New York: Maternity Center Association, 1955.

Mbiti, John S. *African Religions and Philosophy.* New York: Doubleday, 1969.

Medders, Orbie. "Black Grads in Greene Head North." *Birmingham Post Herald,* 7 August 1974, p. 6.

Mongeau, Beatrice, Harvey L. Smith, and Ann Manney. "The "'Granny Midwife': Changing Roles and Functions of a Folk Practitioner." *American Journal of Sociology* 66 (1960): 497–500.

Morton, Julia F. *Folk Remedies of the Low Country.* Miami: E. A. Seemann Publishing, 1974.

Mosley, Franklin S., Mrs., ed. *Snedecor's Greene County Directory 1856.* Reprint, Eutaw: Mrs. Franklin S. Mosley, 1981.

Oliver, Thomas W. " 'King Cotton' in Alabama: A Brief History." *Alabama Heritage* 35 (1995): 16–26.

Onabamiro, Sanya Dojo. *Why Our Children Die: The Causes and Suggestions for Prevention of Infant Mortality in West Africa.* London: Methuen, 1949.

Owen, Thomas McAdory. *History of Alabama and Dictionary of Alabama Biography.* Chicago: S.J. Clarke, 1921. Reprint, Spartanburg: Reprint Company, 1978.

Parker, Jacqueline K., and Edward M. Carpenter. "Julia Lathrop and the Children's Bureau: The Emergence of an Institution." *Social Science Review* 55 (1981): 60–77.

Parsons, Elsie Clews. *Folk-Lore of the Sea Islands, South Carolina.* Chicago: Afro-Am Press, 1969.

Pennington, Estill Curtis. "The Climate of Taste in the Old South." *Southern Quarterly* 24 (1985): 7–31.

Porterfield, Mac. "Negro Demonstrations Ban in Greene County Extended." *Birmingham Post Herald,* 10 September 1965, p. 8.

Priya, Jacqueline Vincent. *Birth Traditions and Modern Pregnancy Care.* Rockport, Massachusetts: Element, 1992.

Rawls, Phillip. "Unlicensed Midwife Faces Charges Again." *Montgomery Advertiser,* 4 March 1994, p. 1.

Reeb, Rene M. "Granny Midwives in Mississippi: Career and Birthing Practices." *Journal of Transcultural Nursing* 4 (1992): 18–27.

Richardson, Elizabeth H., Viola T. Chandler, and Lillian H. Harvey. *Final Report on the Effect of Nursing Care on Selected Aspects of Premature Infant Welfare in the Home.* Tuskegee, Alabama: Tuskegee Institute, 1967.

Robinson, Beverly J. "Life Narratives: A Structural Model for the Study of Black Women's Culture." In *Current Perspectives on Aging and the Life Cycle,* edited by Zena S. Blau, 127–40. Greenwich: JAI Press, 1985.

Rogers, William Warren, Jr. "The Eutaw Prisoners: Federal Confrontation with Violence in Reconstruction Alabama." *Alabama Review* 43 (1990): 98–121.

Rothman, Barbara Katz. *Encyclopedia of Childbearing: Critical Perspectives.* Phoenix, Arizona: Oryx Press, 1993.

Savitt, Todd L. *Medicine and Slavery: The Diseases and Health Care of Blacks in Antebellum Virginia.* Urbana: University of Illinois Press, 1978.

Sikora, Frank. "Greene County's Civil Rights Mark Made 25 Years Ago in Special Vote." *Birmingham News,* 29 July 1994, section 3, p. 1.

———. "Greene Negro Leaders Rap Abernathy-Led Pool March." *Birmingham News*, 12 August 1969, p. 1.

———. "Negro Winners in Greene Will Be Sworn in Aug. 11." *Birmingham News*, 2 August 1969, p. 2.

Singh, Gopal K., and Stella M. Yu. "Infant Mortality in the United States: Trends, Differentials, and Projections, 1950 through 2010." *American Journal of Public Health* 85 (1995): 957–64.

Slaughter, John H. *New Battle over Dixie: The Campaign for a New South*. Dix Hills, New York: General Hall, 1992.

Southern Regional Council. "Crackdown in the Black Belt: On to Greene County." *Southern Changes* 7 (1985): 2–5.

Stoney, George C., and the Georgia Department of Health. *All My Babies*. Distributed by Columbia University Press, 1952.

———. "The Process of Film Making: *All My Babies* Research." In *Film Book I*, edited by Robert Hughes, 79–96. New York: Grove Press, 1959.

Suitts, Steve. "Games Registrars Play." *Southern Changes* 7 (1985).

Susie, Debra Anne. *In the Ways of Our Grandmothers: A Cultural View of Twentieth-Century Midwifery in Florida*. Athens: University of Georgia Press, 1988.

Tart, Ruby Pickens. "Carrie Dykes—Midwife." In *From Hell to Breakfast*, edited by Mody C. Boatright and Donald Day, 21–28. Dallas: Southern Methodist University Press, 1967.

Terry, Paul W., and Verner M. Sims. *They Live on the Land: Life in an Open-Country Southern Community*. 1940. Reprint, Tuscaloosa: University of Alabama Press, 1993.

Thomas, Margaret W. "Social Priority No. 1: Mothers and Babies." *Public Health Nursing* (1942): 442–45.

Thomson, Bailey. "In Greene County: Health Care Clinic Offers Many Aid." *Tuscaloosa News*, 2 February 1975, p. 6.

Tullos, Allen. "Crackdown in the Black Belt: Not-So-Simple Justice." *Southern Changes* (May/June, 1985): 2–10.

Ulrich, Laurel Thatcher. *A Midwife's Tale: The Life of Martha Ballard,*

*Based on Her Diary, 1785–1812.* New York: Alfred A. Knopf, 1990.

U.S. Bureau of the Census. *Housing, 1940.* Vol. 2. Washington: U.S. Government Printing Office, 1943.

Vermeer, Donald E., and Dennis A. Frate. "Geophagia in Rural Mississippi: Environmental and Cultural Contexts and Nutritional Implications." *The American Journal of Clinical Nutrition* 32 (1979): 2129–35.

Walker, Alice. *Revolutionary Petunias and Other Poems.* New York: Harcourt Brace Jovanovich, 1971.

Washington, Booker T. "The Negro Doctor in the South." *The Independent* 63 (1907): 89–91.

Wilson, Freddie Paul. "Medical Care in Greene County," *Alabama Social Welfare* 3 (1938): 13.

Webb, H. Y. Correspondence. Department of Health, State Health Officer Correspondence, 1882–83. Alabama Department of Archives and History.

Weil, Clarence. Brannon, Peter, Correspondence. Alabama Department of Archives and History.

Woodward, C. Vann. *The Strange Career of Jim Crow.* New York: Oxford University Press, 1974.

World Health Organization. "Appropriate Technology for Birth." *The Lancet* 2 (August 1985): 436–37.

Zippert, John. "Greene County." In *Fifteen Years Ago . . . Rural Alabama Revisited,* edited by the U.S. Commission on Civil Rights, 43–52. Clearinghouse Publication 82, December 1983.

# Index

abdominal massage. *See* massage
Abernathy, Ralph T., 114, 119
abortion, 110
activity: postpartum, 42, 49; during labor, 37, 82
African Americans. *See* blacks
African birthing traditions, 40–41, 42, 43
afterbirth: burial of, 40, 41–42, 96; burning of, 96; convulsions and, 105; delivery of, 93–94, 96, 110; examination during midwife training, 73; medicinal plants and, 39; and Mrs. Smith's second child, 48–49; salting of, 41, 42
AIDS, 150
Alabama Board of Health, 67
Alabama Bureau of Maternal and Child Health, 65
Alabama Department of Health: final midwife training conference, 139; funding of state and county health departments, 67
alcohol and consciousness, 103
alum, 110
Anderson, Ella, 5, 70, 75

Andrew Memorial Hospital, Tuskegee: as black hospital, 35–36; care of premature infants, 115; midwife training program, 64–65, 68
apprentice midwives, 44
asafetida bag, 39
ashes, not sweeping, 87
Asian birthing traditions, 41, 42
auction of slaves, 23
automobile, birth in, 105

babies from stumps, 32
back massage, 89. *See also* massage
balm, for female trouble, 110
bamboo briar root, 38, 39, 53
bath: after childbirth, 98; hot, 39, 47, 88–89; medicinal, 40; oil, 40
bearing down, 47; lack of, 108; physical support from midwife, 83
birth certificates, 102, 117
birth control, 47–48
birth fire, 40, 41
birthing pallet, 85; newspaper as, 55, 88

# WOMEN AND HEALTH SERIES

*Rima D. Apple and Janet Golden, Editors*

The series examines the social and cultural construction of health practices and policies, focusing on women as subjects and objects of medical theory, health services, and policy formulation.

---

**Making Midwives Legal:**
*Childbirth, Medicine, and the Law, second edition*
  RAYMOND G. DEVRIES

**The Selling of Contraception:**
*The Dalkon Shield Case, Sexuality, and Women's Autonomy*
  NICOLE J. GRANT

**And Sin No More:**
*Social Policy and Unwed Mothers in Cleveland, 1855–1990*
  MARIAN J. MORTON

**Women and Prenatal Testing:**
*Facing the Challenges of Genetic Technology*
    Edited by KAREN H. ROTHENBERG and
    ELIZABETH J. THOMSON